T0325751

# a
# Paradigm
# of
# Care

# a
# Paradigm
# of
# Care

by

**Robert Stake**

*and*

**Merel Visse**

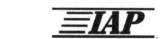

**INFORMATION AGE PUBLISHING, INC.**
Charlotte, NC • www.infoagepub.com

**Library of Congress Cataloging-in-Publication Data**

CIP record for this book is available from the Library of Congress
http://www.loc.gov

ISBNs:   978-1-64802-338-5 (Paperback)

978-1-64802-339-2 (Hardcover)

978-1-64802-340-8 (ebook)

Printed in the United States of America

# CONTENTS

# ACKNOWLEDGMENTS

# IN APPRECIATION

We are grateful to many people who vigilantly and generously
shared their time and thoughts on the manuscript.
To those who—hopefully—will stay in conversation
with us for long times to come.
Thanks to you the manuscript matured into its present form.

Alan Knox, C. Deborah Laughton,
Bob Louisell, Brinda Jegatheesan, Mike Stake,
Sara Stake, Jeff Stake, Yali Feng, Tom Seals, David Jenkins,
Dan McCollum, Charles Cowger, Jacqueline Kool,
Michael Kolen, Ronald Oosterhof,
Truus Teunissen, Paul Lindhout, and all those
who practice a care paradigm, day in, day out.

We especially want to thank Mrs. Osvalda Pellegrini for
allowing us to use
Gino Pellegrini's work on the cover of this book:
Weaving with mixed materials, 224 x 140 cm. Signed, 1982.

**Gino Pellegrini** has long alternated artistic research with scenography, the design and painting of theatrical scenery since he was young and emigrated from Veneto, Italy, to the United States. He studied architecture at UCLA and the University of Southern California and fine arts at the Los Angeles Art Center School. In cinema he worked for the major Hollywood production houses.

After he went back to Italy, his art practice revolved around research and artistic experimentation. He cared for buildings and anonymous or even degraded areas for which beauty seemed a distant mirage. He wanted to work with the grayness and anonymity of neighborhoods, use the references to anthropological and environmental culture that he was able to find there, using materials "found" in different forms—leaves, branches, newspapers. In his environmental scenography he studied the intervention in relation to the subjectivity of the spaces and its users, thus varying the thematic, visual, chromatic, and technical choices according to the different psychological, historical, architectural factors and landscaping. This is one of the reasons why we chose his work on the cover of this book: his capability of creating a world that respects context, community, and openness to the subtleties of the stories of the people who give and receive care.

www.ginopellegrini.it

# INTRODUCTION

## A Paradigm

### Robert Stake and Merel Visse

It is a book of appreciation, partly to you today, a caregiver. Partly to all those who have cared for us all through life and continue to do so. And partly to caregivers and those who receive it around the world during the covid-19 pandemic, and for all time to follow. Even though we know only part of it, we appreciate what you are doing, what you have done, and what you will do in the future to raise the expectations that those in need of care will get it.

This book traces our thoughts since October, 2019. They are thoughts of appreciation. We think of a perception, an attitude, a predisposition, a point of view, a belief, a poetic, a vision, an ethic, a prism: a paradigm. A paradigm is a sweeping, earth-covering, grand way of being, accepted by many people. A care paradigm is a covenant, a set of ideas, claiming that everyone, near and far, should be cared for, protected, treated with dignity, respect, nurtured, and comforted. Some will call it humanistic. Some will call it love. We will call it care. The predisposition exists far and wide, whether named or not. We are using the name paradigm with a purpose, to help emphasize that, in most places, in families and cities and villages, even within both activist and isolationist populations, the private and public commitment to care is, clearly, too narrow now and falling short of the need.

Care hears the moan of indifference. It draws upon the eyes of the heart. Care is about the care humans have for other humans.[1] A paradigm is about how we see the need for care. A care paradigm, the grand beholding, is manifest in how we provide for others, how we nurture them, give succor, how we are disposed, and are not, to sacrifice to relieve their hurt. It is not only caring for those visibly needing care, unable to care for themselves, but caring for all, the living and the surround of living, having a disposition that the hurts, large and small, that all of us carry, arouse concern and relief from and for each individual, the community and the world. It is a carrying on of the appreciation we have today.

## A FIELD OF INQUIRY

Like breathing, much of being human needs care. Individually we have known and given care. Many in great concert. The work of the farmer, the field of agriculture, was devoted to nurturing of selected parts of nature. Medicine, psychology, and education concentrated on control and of the human condition. These helped define our culture, but they did not define human caring. Prenatal caution, preparation for achievement testing, driving lessons, and balanced accounts require being careful but they should not be confused with caring.

Poets and nurses have had a grand history of caring as aspiration and practice. At least briefly, most people have experienced caring, both as givers and receivers. But caring is also a complex phenomenon of society to be studied. Caring is an object of disciplined search and writing. Writers have told of a history of human caring extending back before science and religion (Duby and Perrot, 1992–2004). Long before habits, there was nature, and the nature of humans from whatever beginning was, at times, to be caring, to give of one's own being, of one's own force, the shelter and comfort, the love and the restoration, of life.

Families have life-times of caring. Professionals have careers of caring. It is a way of living, a way of working, a way of being human. But care also is a field of study, for which there are leaders, teachers, writers, researchers and followers, seeking ways to do it better. This field of study is a platform for this book. The ethics of giving care and the propensity or ethic of caring are part of the platform.

The terms, care ethic, care ethics and ethics of care are well used in a few circles. They have been written about, eloquently, by many authors, especially Carol Gilligan, Joan Tronto, Nel Noddings, Virginia Held, and Eva Kittay. The first that many of us heard was feminist writer Carol Gilligan. In her book, *In a Different Voice* (Gilligan, 1982), she addressed the uniqueness of being feminine. She traced differences in moral reasoning between girls and boys. She opened the path for others, extending philosophic thinking about care beyond the field of feminist studies. It became a realization of an ethic of care.

Care studies arrived in volumes in the 1990s. Joan Tronto, in her book *Moral Boundaries* (1993), examined how care ethics might further mature by reviewing the strategy of women's morality and women's sensitivity to care and nurturing. Tronto drew attention to the "limitations" of thinking about care built upon a strongly feminist perspective, and from thinking about morality and politics as distinct. Morality could not go on without politics, and vice versa. They intertwine. Later on, Tronto furthered her argument for care ethics as a political ethic. Care does not only occur in the private realms of our lives but becomes part of public policy and the organization of society. In her book *Caring Democracy* (2013), she put care at the center of how we allocate responsibilities in society as a whole.

Within caregiving, the provocations of dependency and vulnerability were carefully examined by Eva Feder Kittay (1999). Another presence, empathy, runs across this special literature, but Educational Philosopher Nel Noddings (2005) contrasted empathy with a needed deeper understanding, an engrossment of the situation of the recipient, especially for those whose worlds are hard to reach. Her concept of engrossment has become a critique of empathy. Putting care as the very most basic value at the center of moral theory has been the claim of Virgina Held (2005), and connecting it with justice. The feminist philosopher Sarah Ruddick chose to develop care from a traditional source, maternal thinking.

A list here of additional active scholars from a variety of disciplines: Maurice Hamington, Daniel Engster, Fiona Robinson, Carlo Leget, Inge van Nistelrooij, Helen Kohlen, Rachel Adams, Hee-Kang Kim, Elena Pulcini, Sandra Laugier, Frans Vosman♱, Sophie Bourgault, and Alistair Niemeijer. We could add critical sociologists, aestheticsts, program evaluators, educational researchers, and on. Here we have several generations of care ethicists, setting the scene for what has now become an interdisciplinary field of inquiry. And soon, new scholars will appear and enrich the field: promising newcomers such as Maggie Fitzgerald who writes about care ethics as a political ethic and Simon van der Weele doing research on dependency and care. Arts researchers contribute too: Finnish artist Kaisu Koski, based in The Netherlands and the United Kingdom, studied the anti-vaccine movement. And Elena Cologni, a Fellow at the Cambridge School of Art who, together with one of us, founded a network on Art and Care.

Nowadays, care ethics as a field of inquiry is a coming together of philosophers, sociologists, political scientists, and many others (Leget et al., 2017). Their research and scholarship is on care either as a practice, a theory, and an ethic. Alliances abound and reach beyond fields and complexities. The writings show a distinction between the caring sciences as practiced in health care settings, political science and the health and medical humanities, and the field of care ethics and theory. The care ethicists think of care as a central force in the lives of people, of how institutions are structured and of society in general. Here, care serves as an ethic having theory and practice to foster a more just and equitable society. The writings of care ethicists have provided an intellectual foundation for understanding care as a worldview, its relationship to justice, and for the infinite acts of caring, their contextuality and complexity. It is the platform for our book.

These scholars and researchers have been meeting at a variety of conferences and outings.[2] As of this writing, recent and upcoming program topics of interest are ever so many: care and ecology, care and precarity, decolonizing care, care as an epistemology and ontology, care as an anthropology, care and economy, new-materialism and care, care and the distribution of wealth, care in spirituality and religion, care and animals, care and post-humanism, care and performative philosophy, care and poetry, care and aesthetics, and the relationship between theory and empirical research on care.

## THE ZEITGEIST

In this book, we want to give special attention to the literature's contribution to the practical arts of caring, to the heart of it. We want to learn and draw upon all we can from many authors. They have recognized the ethic/paradigm as the construction of understanding of the zeitgeist of care, its spirit, not only the virtue but the need for care-enabling practices. Our task in this book is to join with the reader in stretching that understanding, that Zeitgeist. We will speak at length about the acts of caring and about the heart of care, to broaden the sweep and deepen the flow of the paradigm. The rich palette of literature shows the appeal and broad approach to care.

In this book, we explore care as a pathway to learn about what it means to be a caring human being in contemporary contexts. This could be a phenomenology of care as a creative and deeply human activity that is about concern for the "other." This could be seen as a psychology or an anthropology of the caring human being. We are not so concerned with positioning ourselves in one or more disciplines, nor do we explain much about the lens through which we view care. We are not so concerned about what conceptually constitutes care, to view care as an object for the mind, and, most of the time, we do not aim to dwell on definitions. What we want is to join and enlarge the chorus of caring.

The book is about collective empathy in our society. Magnificent empathy, and inadequate. Each of us has a caring ethic, ever active, ebb and flow, sometimes extending only to those most dear, sometimes fixated mostly on ourselves. At other times and places, generous and generic, extending beyond political and cultural environs, embracing little less than the needs and wants of all creatures.

Naturally, the distress of each creature varies, some with easy respite, some with little hope of respite. It comes and goes, ebbs and flows. Any one complex of grievances is visible against the background of grievances of others, but even so, none to be dismissed by a caring society. Thinking not as one, but of all. Helping individuals, but expecting, moving toward, better care for all. It would be a society that acts in harmony, with compassion as well as reason. That caring society goes beyond its expertise in triage, ranking the wounded according to their injury. It goes beyond a science aimed at naming and correlating their hurts. The caring society energizes an intuition to help all who can draw our hand.

A care paradigm would be, could be, a resonance of the human spirit, an ethic of proportion, a vision of our leaders, a belief of our people, a point of view of our media, a disposition of our children, a shared attitude, a penetrating perception of how people care for and take care of the people they love.

The book is recognition that care is expressed in many ways but is victim to many common definitions of success in homes and purchasings and satellite deliveries. Most personalistic dispositions are pretty much locked in, but we are capable of adjustments and new fascinations. This is not a how-to book, but hopefully it will be persuasion to recognize and foster an expanded caring paradigm.

A few words more about the concept of paradigm. We are thinking of it as idea or spirit, a persuasion both to give and receive care. It is a cultural phenomenon, a sense of reality, a way of living. We also are earth-bound, thinking of paradigm as a cloud or shelter or canopy. For all persons and for each person this paradigm-canopy has a different coverage (see Figure 0.1).

Our image of canopy was enriched by Will McWhinney, who described it in *Grammars of Engagement* (n.d.), an unpublished manuscript, as follows:

> And for ecologists, a canopy describes the roof formed by the great trees of a rain forest that hide the ground from sun and drying winds. The canopy creates an ecology distinct from that on the ground below in the shade of the great trees. This ecology is "groundless" floating fifty to two hundred feet over the forest floor, a tangle of branches and vines inhabited by its own flora, fauna, and phenomena. It is both 'of the earth' and transcends its rules.

This book picks up on the caring to be found in human relationships ever since there have been human relationships. Back then, individuals joined, one on one, not only to propagate and to protect and to adorn

**Figure 0.1**

*Canopy*

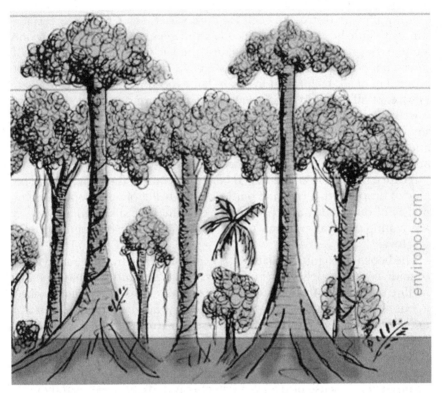

*Source image:* enviropol.com

one another, but to help make life better. They banded together not only to hunt and gather and fight and dance but to help make life better, collectively as well as individually.

And wherever stories were told and books written, there are representations of caring, for babies, for spouses, for fellows, and the infirm. Some stories are of specialists, later called firemen and nurses and chaplains and counselors, and many are of caregivers who have no credentials or rituals but follow their consciences to ease pain and discrimination. We have little shortage of the images of taking care. We have had caves and castles and hospitals and schools and shelters to take care of multiple needs.

Alas, we do it selectively, for those who can pay, for those who "deserve" it, for those who have earned our trust and devotion. We are not so good at searching out the unseen. We are not so good at raising expectations of giving help to those of different color or survival skill or credit rating or smell of sweat. We are not so good at vitalizing a care ethic where it doesn't fit the tryptic.

Naomi Shihab Nye (1995) captured that in these words:

## Kindness

Before you know what kindness really is
you must lose things,
feel the future dissolve in a moment
like salt in a weakened broth.
What you held in your hand,
what you counted and carefully saved,
all this must go so you know
how desolate the landscape can be
between the regions of kindness.
How you ride and ride
thinking the bus will never stop,
the passengers eating maize and chicken
will stare out the window forever.
Before you learn the tender gravity of kindness
you must travel where the Indian in a white poncho
lies dead by the side of the road.
You must see how this could be you,
how he too was someone
who journeyed through the night with plans
and the simple breath that kept him alive.
Before you know kindness as the deepest thing inside,
you must know sorrow as the other deepest thing.
You must wake up with sorrow.
You must speak to it till your voice
catches the thread of all sorrows
and you see the size of the cloth.
Then it is only kindness that makes sense anymore,
only kindness that ties your shoes
and sends you out into the day to gaze at bread,
only kindness that raises its head
from the crowd of the world to say
It is I you have been looking for,
and then goes with you everywhere
like a shadow or a friend.

With appreciation, our book presents a poetics of care that is essentially in and out, up and down, rhythmic, at times discordant. This book may help us connect with the fullness of care, with the heart of care as it sustains us. With this book we hope to gently stretch an intimate space that connects our mutuality. We invite you to consider care in this particular fullness. To seize its reality, its quality, its soul, and to imagine and—in the long run— perhaps to inaugurate a reshaping: a newly revitalized paradigm of care.

## REFERENCES

Duby, G., & Perrot, M. (Eds.). (1992–2004). *A history of women in the West* (5 vols.). Harvard University Press.

Gilligan, C. (1982). *In a different voice: Psychological theory and women's development.* Harvard University Press.

Held, V. (2005). *The ethics of care.* Oxford University Press.

Kittay, E. F. (1999). *Love's labor. Essays on women, equality, and dependency.* Routledge.

Leget, C., van Nistelrooij, I., & Visse, M. (2017). Beyond demarcation: Care as an interdisciplinary field of inquiry. *Nursing Ethics.* https://doi.org/10.1177/0969733017707008

McWhinney, W. (n.d.). *Grammars of engagement* (Unpublished manuscript). University of Los Angeles.

Noddings, N. (2005). An ethic of care. In A. Cudd & R. Andreasen (Eds.), *Feminist theory: A philosophical anthology* (pp. 251–263). Blackwell.

Shihab Nye, N. (1995). *Words under the words: Selected poems* (A Far Corner Book). The Eighth Mountain Press.

Tronto, J. (1993). *Moral boundaries: A political argument for an ethic of care.* Routledge.

Tronto, J. (2013). *Caring democracy: Markets, equality and justice.* New York University Press.

1. National Domestic Workers Alliance; Family Caregiver Alliance; National Center on Caregiving.
2. Such as the International Care Ethics Research Consortium Conferences (www.care-ethics.org) and initiatives like Caring #4 by the New Alphabet School in collaboration with M.1 Arthur Boskamp-Stiftung in June 2020.

# CHAPTER 1

# EQUITY AND
# SOCIAL DISTANCE

A paradigm is a sweeping, grand feeling, accepted widely by people. A care paradigm is an agreement that people, near and far, should be cared for, protected, treated with dignity and respect, nurtured, and comforted and emboldened in spirit. We call it various things, humanism, Christianity, charity, love. Whatever. For including all such benevolences, we are using the name *paradigm*. The magnitude helps emphasize that in most places, even in families and remote villages and out to activist groups and philanthropies, the broad commitment to care is, today, falling short.

Even as appreciative of what you do, we will speak at length about extending the feeling of caring beyond the present location and range. We all, mostly all, deserve prizes for caring for some in the family, and some in the neighborhood, and generosity in giving to the Red Cross, food banks, and victims of refugee camps. Seriously. But our eyes are shuttered, partly by solicitations in the mail, partly by the exposure of scams, partly by our fears of being taken in.

## MANIPULATION

We learned what it was like to be "locked-down" and "self-quarantined." We learned what it was like to keep a few feet from other people. The pandemic has changed our lives. It was the most powerful new phenomenon that

*a Paradigm of Care*, pp. 1–11
Copyright © 2021 by Information Age Publishing
All rights of reproduction in any form reserved.

"our" world had experienced. Greater than Brexit, greater than social media, greater than climate change and wind power, greater than resistance to immigration. We have only a small idea how much it changed, how much it still will change, our lives.

As of now we might guess that it will erode trust in governments. For many, trust had long worn thin, but hundreds of thousands are dying because short-sighted leaders around the world failed to heed warnings about potential pandemics. Perhaps never again will employment, work with a paycheck, be available to half the people. Perhaps the availability of tropical fruit 'round the year will not be common. Home owning may become quaint. It seems there are new surprises ahead. Trust might become one of the shortest supplies.

We have seen a diminishing supply of privacy. What we plan to do, what we plan to buy, where we have thoughts of going, is already in the cloud. What reason have we to believe that something will happen that will protect our communication, our movement, our secrets? We are laid bare. And this is not the apex of the curve. It too is exponential. We may develop some powers to keep our intimacies to ourselves. But the devices of the intruders, the manipulators, yes, the *1980* thought police, are likely to be better, more clever, more penetrating, than the curtains and masks and coveralls we can devise. Perhaps we will get used to exposure.

Mobilization for protection requires a sense of common purpose. It seems we have it, but we have had common purpose all of the 21st Century, and we could not see how to achieve protection, safety, and care. It perhaps is wrong to think that we need to agree on what do we seek in common before developing it. It is often implied that in order for the journey to succeed we have to agree on the destination. That is often implied by those opposing the journey, those selling tickets, and those writing blogs, knowing that we will not agree. In this book, we will move ahead without blue-printing the means and the ends of a caring paradigm. We will hope for some shared feelings.

Mobilization for protection requires a reservoir of energy. We will not be thinking of the energy of a protest march. We will not be thinking of the energy of a political campaign, such as the energy of the Tea Party or of Occupy Wall Street. It may be what mainly drives the Me-Too movement. The energy we seek already exists in the caring to be found in almost every family, the bondedness, the love, the sacrifice. It exists in prenuptials, in team loyalties.

It is a reservoir greater than the watersheds of the rivers of the world. Some of the energy could spin off, some of it could swell and pop out. The spirit of brotherhood/sisterhood, motherhood/fatherhood is already concocted for caring. It is already doing immense good. It mobilized for Diana. It mobilized for Gandhi. We hope that the stories we tell, and the chuckles we might draw, and the reminiscences we provoke, with your help, may release more from that reservoir.

Who to help, what to do, when and where is up to you. We will talk about some folks up close, and some neighbors (fahrbors?) in Tijuana and Dhaka. Close and far. We will try to make the reading worth your time. But if it is already time to close the book and call grandma, do that.

## SOCIAL DISTANCE

We each need help in deciding how to be helpful to those many others close to our visions of decent living. Really close. How can we measure that closeness? Not long ago, well, actually, a hundred years ago, sociologist Emory Bogardus (1947) devised a scale for indicating people's willingness to be close to people, including members of diverse racial and ethnic groups. Here are seven steps on the scale:

- As close as relatives by marriage (i.e., legal spouse of a close relative) (score 1.00)
- As my close personal friends (2.00)
- As neighbors on the same street (3.00)
- As co-workers in the same occupation (4.00)
- As citizens in my country (5.00)
- As non-citizen visitors in my country (6.00)
- Would *exclude* from entry into my country (7.00)

These steps may not be sufficiently uniform for some sociological research, but they help us repeat the understanding that we care more deeply for those within six feet and less deeply for those quite different from us. You did not need Bogardus to tell you what you knew already. Close is close.

And we should not be urged to care for everyone the same. That would be nonsense. And we should not be expected to have good reasons for whom we care. But we could rethink the question how to extend more and better care to lots of people somewhat like us—without asking too much, without threatening our limited savings. And we would expect that it would mean to learn more about the situations of those with needs. That is partly what this book is about, the practices and contexts out to which we should extend care. We will not try to tell you how; we do not know your situation. But exploring the concept of care in the many contexts of care, we might free up more of your generosities.

## EQUITY

Each of us has the power to grant privilege. Our smiles and attention help make other lives better. With carelessness and misperception, we make other lives poorer. Collectively our social action makes life more livable for some children, and less livable for others.

To be rational about values is at the heart of research on ethics, where it is generally taken that rights, respect, and privilege should be distributed equally to all. But for various purposes, including survival, legality, and personal preference, the distribution will often be unequal, often extraordinarily unequal. In his *Theory of Justice,* John Rawls (1971) started by recognizing that privilege can seldom be distributed equally, or justice equally served. He argued that errors should fall to the benefit of the least advantaged.

> When they were younger, both Tomas and his wife Marie worked. Then came the children. They still needed Marie's wages to pay the bills. Tomas would make more if promoted, but to get a promotion would mean working overtime. Marie felt the children needed more from their father.

There are diverse and competing ways of being rational. To think through a matter deeply is not necessarily a heading toward equity. It is easy to get side-tracked.

Strongly influenced by Rawls, philosophers Ernest House and Kenneth Howe (1999) published *Values in Education and Social Research.* They urged that researchers and others promote democratic values even to the point of setting up formal deliberation on issues developed in their quests. Democratic evaluation was created by Barry MacDonald (1993) and others (Green, 2016; Simons, 1987) to prioritize issues particularly of public interest in government-funded projects. Its designs are inclusive of issues recognized by government agencies and other funders, but quietly advocate a public need to know. House and Howe constrained themselves to recognition of what the public should know but went on to advocate facilitating dialogue among the various sides. While Rawls concentrated on sensitivity during interpretation, a silent advocacy, House and Howe would make the advocacy more open to view.

A banner across the top of the great seal of the state of Nebraska is emboldened with the words, Equality before the Law. The same motto is associated with Article 7 of the Universal Declaration of Human Rights and other documents. They are associated with a reform in English law to constrain favorable treatment given people of privilege. The words are mainly interpreted as meaning each citizen shall be treated as having the same rights when facing legal proceedings. Treat all the same. The original

**Figure 1.1**

*Equality Before the Law*

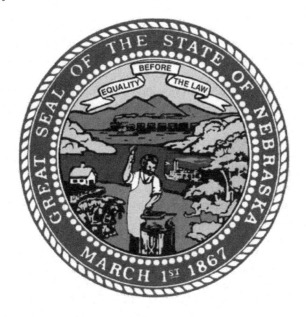

intent seems not quite "to be fair," not that much reform, but at least to be more uniform.

Equality before the law is now widely interpreted as assuring the same treatment and that that legal treatment will be fair. It could do more for fairness. The motto might be interpreted as meaning more fair than legally fair. "Before" sometimes means "in priority over." Your entry before mine. Your care before mine. Equality before the law could mean that each is to be treated fairly *before* legal regard and even without obeisance to what is considered equal. Equitable instead of equal.

Reparations sometimes will be made in the name of equity. Equity could be taken to mean making adjustments to correct inequality. Equality before the law is often interpreted as requiring exactly the same treatment—but "before the law" could be interpreted as meaning that *the situation*, with attention to personal characteristics such as race, gender, color, ethnicity, religion, and disability shall be considered first, in the ways the laws will be interpreted, in order that more equal treatment in the future may be assured. Personal characteristics will not be equal, but interpretation of the law needs to strive toward equality. Equality before the law.

The law does not exist without interpretation of the law. Whether speaking of what the law requires or what the law provides, its meaning depends on interpretation. In its exercise of care, the law requires food service licenses and provides for safe streets. There is no way every bar and every street can be treated exactly the same. Interpretations will vary. The court system exists because the law needs human interpretation. Judges will interpret the law, instructing juries and advocates, who themselves will make their own interpretations, not only of acts being adjudicated, but of the law itself. Whether this is good or bad, it is the way it is. The law is meaningful only in terms of its human interpretations.

Some laws are bad. Drug use laws and campaign finance laws and social media regulations greatly need repair. Reform is difficult. Some legislators strive to write laws of fair treatment and others strive to give preferential treatment. Even the best laws are weak guarantees of equal treatment. Laws are a necessary part of our societal processes and need to be obeyed—partly in our effort to be caring of others—and need to be improved.

People are different. Old and young, rich, and poor, if treated the same, some will be mistreated. Optimum treatment will seldom be identical treatment for all. What appears to be equal treatment may be unfair. Even with meticulous judges, uniform sentencing will yield some bad sentences. Even with fair-minded teachers, some student grades will be more hurtful than helpful. Equality before the law is not good enough.

Equity is a better aspiration. Fairness. Not impartiality, but a limited partiality in the direction of care for those most needing care. Justice. A taking into consideration the effects of the judgment. A recognition of past injustice. A reparation. Not a uniform code of past wrongs and present needs, but a broad weighing of the circumstances, an adjudication.

Of course, no treatment of life for the individual or for the community can be made without a literature, perhaps to include the law and codified experience and Great Books and more. A paradigm of care calls for our predisposition to dig out existing knowledge—for each context—of what is good and bad, and to identify the choices of action and presence of mind that are collectively thought to move things toward higher quality. Equity before the law.

## COMPARISON

The search for quality in the world of Education is exercised by teacher judgment and standardized testing. Clearly the testing and teaching in our schools favor some youngsters more than others. Many students are treated fairly much of the time, others often unfairly. In schools everywhere, *fairness* has not been the highest priority. Poor performance is discriminated against. Teachers prefer to teach children and adults similar to themselves. Parents *want* discrimination that may enhance their children's college and employment opportunities. Privilege is protected by putting down the less privileged.

Standardized tests are the high technology of student comparisons. They sort students into ranks. They do not tell what a student knows. They do not tell what a student can do. No, they do not. They do no more than compare students, one to others, on a hypothetical scale. Many of the tests claim to measure aptitude. In fact, they measure neither intellectual function, nor accomplishment nor potential. Okay, it is true: in diverse groups, they provide scores that "correlate" with *some* brain function, *some* accomplishment, and *some* human potential. Some uses of the tests have been validated, but the consequences of this discrimination reflect public and professional aspirations more than the search for equity in our society.

In scholastic testing, there are winners and losers. No equity is intended. A few test takers step ahead to special privilege, many do not. It is easy for an unthinking world to suppose that scoring will be neutral—helpful more than hurtful. But easy for a thinking person to conclude that being told over and over, "You are inferior," is damaging. Children in schools know their place. So, what is "quality of life" surrounded by people repeatedly lowering expectations of you?

Harvard College has taken the position that, without diversity, "Harvard would lose a great deal of its vitality and intellectual excellence and that the quality of the educational experience offered all students, would suffer" (Counsel for Amicus Curiae, n.d.). Understanding *is* facilitated by diverse perspectives. Diversity *is* catalyst to a healthy society.

Is there need to discriminate among students? Do we need to compare as much as we do? A great deal of thinking involves comparison, that is, of thinking in general. We talk about living, and about ethics, about caregiving, with attention to function, and problematics, and context,—and often we compare with other modes of living and ethics and caregiving. We, Merel and Bob, are persuaded that it is impossible to think, without comparing.

We spend a lot of time comparing people. And it sometimes means putting some people on pedestals and putting other people down. We compete, partly to appear better than we are. We, your authors here, do not suppose we as a people could compete less, or compare less, to think less of what is better and what is inferior. But we wonder if we could be less hurtful. It is hurtful to say that Steven is a slow learner. It is hurtful to report that Samantha had a grade point average of 1.4. Some such stereotyping is inevitable, but not all of it. In school we compare students unnecessarily. It seldom helps a youngster to know that he or she is at the top again. It regularly hurts students to be shown that they are near the bottom again and again.

A teacher needs to know how well a child has performed earlier, and how well classes are progressing, but it does not help a teacher or a child or a society to memorialize scholastic rankings.

There is a passion for knowing who is better and which is best. Comparison thrives in business, politics, sports, and science. But comparison thrives also in child rearing and leisure and education. In required courses, comparison of one person against others, is a problem. If the child has no choice of being there, comparison is an indicator of lack of care.

## DIVERSITY AND INTERSECTIONALITY

With reason and deliberation, law schools and other institutions of higher education closely compare, each against others, the applicants to their programs. The Admission Committees have used a number of criteria for selection of future students, one of them being race. The Indiana School of Law (Bloomington) has also regularly used "geography, viewpoint, undergraduate school and field of study, work and graduate school experience, participation in community services and campus life, economic background, potential for service to the profession, military service, and ethnicity" (Counsel for Amicus Curiae, n.d.).

The School's aim was stated as providing "the highest quality education possible in order to serve the professional community and legal client base in Indiana" As did other law schools and associations, in 2002 the Indiana school filed a brief (Counsel for Amicus Curiae, n.d.) in the U.S. Supreme Court supporting the 1978 Bakke case (*University of California Regents vs. Bakke*, 1978) decision that allowed consideration of race among other factors. How law is taught depends on who the students are. The Indiana brief quoted a law student claiming:

> Being confronted with opinions from different socioeconomic and ethnic realms forces you to develop logical bases for the opinions you have and to discard those not based on such logic. You simply are forced to think more critically about your opinions when you know that people with differing opinions are going to ask you to explain yourself. (Orfield & Whitla, 2001)

Life is diverse around the world, and complex. Sections of each life are recognizable within the diversity. Some personal characteristics—such as race, age, test performance, military service, gender, congeniality, also "lawyering potential,"—are sections scrutinized by admissions committees. Similarly, such sections are differentially viewed by all of us, often causing too simple a view. We all belong to many stereotypes. Long ago, Walter was the baker in a segregated army company, and reminded by a recently-arrived helper, in a relaxed moment, that "You White guys all look the same."

To counter the stereotyping, new approaches to diversity have emerged. Some writings call it "intersectionality" (Hankivsky, 2014). As an equity point of view, intersectionality rejects the prioritization of any order of categories. Intersectionality can be thought of as the uniqueness of any overlap of circles in a Venn diagram, the circles in a Balantine ale ad. Or triangles or hexagons. Intersectionality does not just add categories (race + class + gender) (*University of California Regents vs. Bakke,* 1978). It considers cases as a special group when each share multiple traits, such as all the poor Caribbean women. It is a complex pattern, a quilt of meaning, recognizing the complex life of each of us, never symmetrical, always multisplendored. Caring dares not treat people simply, because it will miss the regular heartbeat or the occasional stabbing of enduring life. A simple flower or strumming guitar needs not be intersectional but the beholding of someone or some peoples as no more than the stereotype is not a suitable way of treating them. A health club or nursing-home policy risks treating too many people as undifferentiated.

Care gets stereotyped as something done mostly by women. Elderly women are especially stereotyped. Grandmas, more than you and us, we will argue, become uniquely deprived of many of the joys and satisfactions of earlier experience. Grandpa is gone, one way or another. With good fortune, grandmas are supported by families and buddies, but forced still to find new activities and satisfactions. In Chapter 8 we present a scene from the south of China. As in our other stories in these chapters, we are reminded of how caring reaches people and of how important it is (is it not for everyone?) to have a caring surround.

For the last few years in many Western countries such as the UK and The Netherlands, social policies reformed quickly. For the Netherlands, this meant the start of a new, locally-oriented care-allocation system within which citizens are held responsible to look after and care for each other. Only citizens lacking resources for care, qualify for aid for professional help. This transition impacted the lives of many people: caretakers and recipients. People who live with an illness or disability and who request assistance with activities such as cleaning their house, are visited by an "advisor" from the local government. The advisor determines *if,* and *what* care will be provided. Informally, these visits are called "Kitchen Table Conversations." Here is an experience of Jacqueline Kool at one of the Conversations:

## KITCHEN TABLE CONVERSATION[1]

By law, advisors urge their "clients" to be self-reliant, asking their family or friends for assistance. Jacqueline has had several of those conversations. She says: *"The outcome of this conversation is always focused on the reduction of costs."* She quotes from the letter that announced the visit: *"You are obliged to cooperate. When we cannot reach you at the aforementioned day and time, this will have consequences for the assistance that you receive."* This tone of voice startles and intimidates her. On the day of the visit, she can barely manage her nerves.

Jacqueline is wheelchair-bound. She politely answers the advisor's questions about her capability to clean her house: *"Yes, I suffer from a chronic, progressive disease, I cannot vacuum my house. It has been like this for the last eight years, and I still cannot do that. As you know, I suffer from a progressive disease."*

Advisor: *"You cannot vacuum, but couldn't you dust your windowsill? You cannot put a bedsheet into the washing machine, but couldn't you put your socks in there? Can you change your bedsheets?"* "No, someone else does that for me," Jacqueline answers.

*"How often do you change your bedsheets? Would neighbors or family be able to help out more?"* Jacqueline: *"I live in a residential care house where everyone is chronically ill or has severe disabilities. We are already doing the most we can."*

Governments aim to reduce costs and urge people to care for one another, but they forget those who would and want to, but who cannot do more. Governments send advisors to re-indicate care (re-evaluate it). Jacqueline: *"All this time spent by advisors to re-evaluate and re-indicate can better be spent on giving us the help that we need. My cleaner costs 20 dollars an hour; these visits of advisors cost double or even triple. A waste of time and money, and precious energy."*

Jacqueline has a cousin, Elsbeth. Elsbeth is 60 years young, was married to a surgeon, lived in a fancy neighborhood until she fell severely ill. Now, she lives in a small apartment, needs financial support. She is on oxygen 24 hours a day and depends on a wheelchair. At first sight, she is someone who does not really live up to the ideal view of an independent citizen: she is without a job, does not have children, is not economically independent. But in practice, her role is indispensable. Every day, she assists the children of her neighbors from North-Africa with their homework, doing math, showing them how to paint and how to play. The other day, Mohammed brought her a box of chocolates to express his gratitude. Despite his dyslexia, she helped him pass his driving exam. For another neighbor who cannot write and read, she takes care of the tax returns. She also knows who is sick, who needs groceries, and who just needs a conversation or chitchat. But for Elsbeth this is normal. It is just what you do: "Nonsense, I just love children. Mohammed helped me with the Christmas tree the other day, so kind. He also fixed my kitchen table."

It is hard to imagine how a world ravaged by pandemic and chafing under quarantine will step forward in its commitment to care. Employment does have to be restored. Economic forces will demand that pockets and promises be dumped for restocking the global market shelves. Will the best of the Kitchen Tables be outmaneuvered by the manipulations of the ad-driven media? Is there a technology that will serve a care paradigm? What could we do to make Amazon care more? Ten chapters from now will not bring us answers, but we need to think deeply about the shortcomings of care right now (whenever right now is). Let us try a chapter entitled "Responsiveness and Ethical Demand" with two more examples of the holistics of care.

## REFERENCES

Bogardus, E. S. (1947). Measurement of personal-group relations. *Sociometry, 10*(4), 306–311.

Counsel for Amicus Curiae (n.d.). *Brief for Indiana University as Amicus Curiae Supporting Respondents*. Curiae Press.

Greene, J. (2016). Advancing equity: Cultivating and evaluation habit. In S. Donaldson & R. Picciotto (Eds.), *Evaluation for an equitable society* (pp. 49–66). Information Age Publishing.

Hankivsky, O. (2014). Rethinking care ethics: On the promise and potential of an intersectional analysis. *The American Political Science Review, 108*(2), 252–264.

House, E., & Howe, K. R. (1999). *Values in evaluation and social research*. SAGE.

MacDonald, B. (1993). A political classification of evaluation studies in education. In M. Hammersley (Ed.), *Social Research—Pphilosophy, politics and practice* (pp. 105–109). SAGE.

Orfield, G., & Whitla, D. (2001). Diversity and legal education: Student experience in leading law schools. In G. Orfield & M. Kurlander (Eds.), *Diversity challenged: Evidence on the impact of affirmative action* (pp. 143–174). Harvard Education Press.

Rawls, J. (1971). *Theory of justice*. Harvard University Press

Simons, H. (1987). *Getting to know schools in a democracy, The politics and process of evaluation*. The Falmer Press.

University of California Regents versus Bakke, 438 U.S. 265 (1978).

## NOTE

1. Based on Jacqueline Kool's article in the Dutch NRC Newspaper, titled: *Keukentafelgesprek is zeer vernederend*. January, 9, 2015.

# CHAPTER 2

# RESPONSIVENESS AND THE ETHICAL DEMAND

For four years, Keith Lane spent his days patrolling an eight mile stretch of coastline, spotting people who might jump. During those years, Keith prevented 25 people from taking their lives. To him, this was neither duty nor obligation. His commitment appeared from empathy. "I sat where you sat, I know where you are." Although people believe that they have the right to take their own life, Keith believes that people "can get over it." He wants them to have a second chance and stops them from "going over." Years earlier, Keith's wife had committed suicide by jumping off the cliff. Helping others and keeping coming back to the cliff has been a mission for him (Lane, 2014)

## ETHICAL DEMAND

Sometimes, a care ethic crosses our path unforeseen. In those instances, care is more than just an invitation. It is a call not to be ignored. Indifference is not an option. We are pulled by a force that urges us to act. An ethical demand (Logstrøp, 1997), perhaps. Its pull is strong and is directed toward someone or something. When this happens, we may wonder "Why me?" But it usually stays silent. No answer. It is just you. No one else takes the responsibility. No one else to rely upon. Think about the parent who gets up at night to comfort a crying child. Or the nurse whose shift ended long ago, but who spends time with her patient because it needs be.

Unfamiliar strangers can call for care. Keith answered that call. He was touched, something was stirred within him that made him want to protect strangers from giving up. By responding, "the other" is affected in turn. This twofold process makes us "come to life." Both people are transformed. Here, a care paradigm helps us come *alive*. This aliveness makes the world more real. Care is linked to the real world: our bodies, our conversations, our institutions, our planet. Care is related to its beginnings and endings. Keith knows this: he senses what is happening on the verge of life and death. On the verge, he knows what it feels like to be in pain, to suffer. He also knows what it means to be alive.

## GOOD AND POOR CARE

To care "well" is about being in relation. We cannot *not* be in relation. We always are. Accepting that we depend on each other and that we are free at the same time. Although care is not inclined to confine or coerce, there can be situations and crises where gentle force is required. Without forces, gentle or wearying, care is nowhere. Strong forces, to be sure, can endanger care and do moral harm. Every parent knows that too much protection may lead to recalcitrance or anger. Too little may lead to chaos. Balanced care can be raw and gentle and firm as a creative force molding and holding, yes, molding and holding.

A person's life, our personal ecosystem: we hold it in our hands. Not always in control, we are not separated from life. We are entangled and bound by our humanity. By holding life in our hands, and letting others hold ours, we take care. But little is said (or fixed) as to *how* this care is to be done. We often care poorly. Care is imbalanced. We all too wearily remember those who need care the most: children without parents, people hungry, those living with a chronic illness and disability. Care is diminished by thinking that we know what others want or need. Some get their needs met, many do not.

Let us go back to Keith. A memorial to Keith's wife was placed on the clifftop. One day, the City Council announced that research had found memorials at the spot could influence people in a distressed state. It removed the memorial from the cliff to "help safeguard lives." The Council supposed it was taking good care of people. But for Keith, this was substituting one lack of care for another. It raised his moral distress. He found it misplaced, insensitive. Keith was given no notice that the cross for his wife would be removed. It was done without his consent. "I was devastated. Although it is time for me to move on, it's my decision when

I want to remove it. If they'd had the decency and compassion to have contacted me, I would have removed it myself."

Often good care and poor care will be mixed together. People have competing ideas about what should be done. So do car companies and NATO allies. Each has a mix of ideas to apply, and some are good and some not so much. The following case from India reminds us of how people living side by side can value life quite differently. It was reported by University of Washington ethnographer Brinda Jegatheesan (2019).

In 2012 during an ethnographic study of attitudes toward cows among native people in South India, I was in the same town as my parents' plantation. Our family cow, named Sita, had recently given birth and was very ill. She was crying frequently and appeared to be comforted by her newborn calf. Dr. Peter (a U.S.-educated veterinarian, a native of India, and a practicing Christian), whose services my parents had utilized for a long time, visited the plantation every two days to treat Sita. Despite the treatments, Sita's condition worsened. Eventually, Dr. Peter informed my father that the cow was in pain and suffering and was convinced that she had at most two months to live. To relieve the cow of her pain and suffering, I suggested euthanasia—to the shocking disbelief of the doctor. He told me that it was an "unthinkable act" and refused to do it. He repeatedly told me that it was a sin to euthanize a cow and that it would be bad karma for him. He also warned me of the karmic repercussions for me as a person of the Hindu faith. Even an offer to pay higher fees did not convince him. The other veterinarians in town also refused my request for euthanasia. Sita died 42 days later. Dr. Peter is a Christian who eats beef and does not identify with the cow as a Hindu does. His attitude toward the cow was profoundly influenced by the prevailing beliefs associated with the sanctity of the cow and the karmic consequences to him, even if he had euthanized the suffering animal for humane reasons.

We will speak more about care of animals in Chapter 9. The mix of care can miss the needs and wants. Society sets the standards and offerings of care. But some care, by others who give, opposes our needs. Just as with the City Council, it is not always clear what the demand for care requires. It may mean moving from thoughtlessness to being directed by compassion and attention. The local Council should have reached out to Keith. Someone from the Council should have put himself out there, taking the risk to connect with what matters to Keith. To care appropriately, someone from the Council could have been attentive to Keith's needs.

## BEING RESPONSIVE

Care as a space for listening and being responsive to and present for another person, is steered by kindness and love. But entering and occupying spaces of caring, by oneself or with others, can also be confusing, threatening, frightening. These experiences can be invisible and difficult to grasp. Tensions lie between good and bad, beautiful and ugly, care and intrusion. When one cares or receives care, differences between different worlds come into contact and, when or where, conflict. Some differences have small impact, others severe. For example, in our vulnerability, in our trajectory, we may like it when our pillow is plumped out a little more, so it supports our back just right, but someone—someone with good intentions—plumps it too hastily, and our needs are not met. When someone's care falls short, we must navigate our disappointment. Perhaps it was the "right" response, but revealing obligation, thus feeling icy, absent genuine, intentional empathy.

> Tomas and Marie have had a good life, with children and friends who make them proud. They don't often talk about the future. Tomas mentioned death, their death, once. Marie looked at him, got up and left the room.

Here, *responsiveness* may be an epistemic or moral virtue that needs cultivation. Responsiveness assists us in learning to "know" the other by practicing receptivity and openness to the experiences of the other: Not by putting yourself in the position of the other, but by considering the position as the other expresses it. One is engaged from the standpoint of the other, but not under the assumption that the other is like the self (Welz, 2015). The distance between the self and the other can never be overcome, but self and other grow into a relationship. Some dub this relationship between the self and other a "third pole" that engages both people (van Nistelrooij, 2014). Others refer to intersubjectivity, and in other contexts some speak of friendship and love. With Bernhard Waldenfels (2016) and Maurice Merleau-Ponty (1994), we imagine this space as an Inter-World. A space where we can dwell in language and that which goes beyond language.

Responding means answering, when given an offering, a challenge, a situation needing attention. We address the persons or problems in this situation, taking aim, moving toward something, going somewhere, perhaps with hope and expectation. It is a hope of caring for someone or something, to better the situation. Not all calls for care make us want to respond. Sometimes nothing happens. But when a call does resonate, we are faced with something that not only makes an effect but addresses us personally. A relationship is established.

## BALANCED SUSPENSION

Who should do what for whom, why, and when? Can we even think about care in such a way? As soon as we care or receive care, we find ourselves in an intricate play. We are interdependent, we are "nested" in relationships: there is a tension between being dependent and free at the same time. One response could be to try to resolve these tensions, to reduce our dependencies, cut people off by regulatory control. Many institutions are focused on controlling those tensions by developing guidelines, rules, and systems-based regulations, all cast in terms of a management rationality. Another route follows the wisdom of less control. Tensions can have structural and creative value for us as human beings, just because they hold us in place, perhaps in balanced suspension, even if only for now, for careful exploration. We move toward being interdependent forms in the spaces of caring. Our interdependence is necessary for solidarity, community, and trust. When the "less-control" view is held, new spaces to care may be found.

Less control also means more time for care to unfold. Care should not be hurried. To care responsively is to "linger with," to understand the importance of being-with the other—of sharing time (Waldenfels, 2016). Some speak of a "tender attentive slowness" (Cixous, 1991). and patience that aids in our approach towards care. Waldenfels (2016) would perhaps add "delay" as in a kind of belated response. That happens to us when we relate to another in situations of care but appearing to us as coming too early. For example, when I am not expecting the story to take a particular turn. Or when I hope for one happening, and something completely different unfolds. Delay can also be a conscious choice, an act of resistance against purposes of appropriation, so dominant in our world today. Care for others may mean caring for delay and slowness. The City Council could have waited a while, just to give Keith some space and to learn more about what occurred there on the cliff. Thus, a balanced suspension of control, of outcomes to reach or—in any important inquiry—of drawing conclusions that may not be the right ones but that are forced upon us.

## LOVING CARE

Let us go back to Keith for another moment. Helping others was healing for him. But there was something else. Actually, there was *someone* else. A few years after his wife committed suicide, Keith met his current wife. Keith says that her love gives him the strength to help others. Here, love is not the same as care, but care can be loving. Some care ethicists speak of *loving care* (van Heijst, 2011). For many of us, "love" usually evokes romantic and erotic tones. For Keith and his wife, love may mean that both are being a witness to the other: getting up in the morning, going out, coming back home, sharing a dinner, and ending the day. Their love may be romantic and erotic, we do not know, but from their story we learn that they support one another when living from "their own center." They also do things for each other: their love translates into actions. Here, Keith's care for strangers means love in a broad sense: neighborly love (agape). It is a response to a demand to love the other without reservations, without expecting anything in return. This kind of love demands generosity, and sometimes sacrifice, but it is altruistic. Otherwise we would not call it neighborly love.

Some say this is mercy, showing the other a shadow of goodness. It is not about what Keith gives, but *that* he gives. The persons he meets at the cliff are absorbed in their suffering, and Keith is drawn by that absorption. He cannot take their place. Anyone who has been a witness to someone in suffering, knows that we feel it in our body when we see another person in pain. We feel it in our heart or belly. But why did Keith, who may have felt this too, stay and act, why did he not run away, why was the suffering of the people he encountered, not too much for him? He may have identified with them because Keith knows what it is like to feel depressed. He may also have acted, because he feels connected with a higher source that steered him to do so. A nonreligious reason would simply be the reciprocity we have as human beings, our mutuality, because we partake in each other's lives. Perhaps it is because his wife loves him, gives to him, that makes it possible for him, in turn, to give to others. This is not unfamiliar in society in general: there are many examples of people who begin charity work because someone else was good to them without wanting anything in return. Love is giving, and love is a gift.

## WE "HAPPEN" TO CARE

Keith was being moved too: figuratively and literally. Not by obligation or social convention, but by a "being-with," as sociologist Zygmunt Bauman (2003) sometimes put it. Bauman made a distinction between being-aside, as an intentional joining together of humans alongside one another; being-with, caused by accidental circumstance in which each human continues to pursue his own purposes; and being-for, because of coincidence and authenticity, not because of choice. Sometimes people just "happen" to care. When it would be a choice, we think we know something about the other, which we may not. This "happening" may be evoked by a call: we respond to the call, without thinking about it. If we start to ask ourselves "why?" then our response, our caring, loses its authenticity. Some think that people are mostly indifferent to each other, that they feel at a distance. When we read the major newspapers, we may believe them impersonal. But there are many people who are concerned about each other, even strangers. In health care, in education.

The primatologist Frans de Waal's (2008) research argues that the basic stance of animals is altruïsm, not indifference, as many economists assert. We have a deep-rooted predisposition for having feelings for others. There are many examples of people who give to others, not to get something back, but because they happen to care. It may be a happening out of the blue, it may come from somewhere else.

Circumstances change, and our caring is drawn differently. This is true in international relations just as much as in personal relations. Strangers become friends; friends become estranged. Social distance expands and contracts. Allies become enemies, and then allies again. In the novel, *1984*, three nations seem to take turns being the victim of the other two (Orwell, 1949). Caring should not be so fickle. Yes, the grounds for our assistance do change, and we ourselves change as well.

In 1864, President Abraham Lincoln chose to begin the Civil War, North against secessionist South. Slavery was not the issue. He acted to preserve the Union. The casualties ultimately passed 600,000 soldiers, on battle-fields and prison camps. What was cared for the most?

In 1945, President Harry Truman approved the atomic bombing of Hiro-shima, Japan to force an end to World War II. Casualties were estimated at over 200,000. He said he thought of those already killed, those who would die with the bombing, and those still to die without it. Was the caring misplaced?

In 1948, after World War II, after picturing Germans and Japanese as rapa-cious and genocidal, Americans created the Marshall Plan to re-establish the economies of their former enemies. Were these careless inconsistencies?

We conclude this chapter with an experience of someone who cared. It is the story of Gate A-4, told by the American-Palestinian poet Naomi Shihab Nye. It goes:

### Gate A-4

Naomi Shihab Nye

Wandering around the Albuquerque Airport Terminal, after learning my flight had been delayed four hours, I heard an announcement: "If anyone in the vicinity of Gate A-4 understands Arabic, please come to the gate im-mediately." Well—one pauses these days. Gate A-4 was my own gate. I went there. An older woman in full traditional Palestinian embroidered dress, just like my grandma wore, was crumpled to the floor, wailing. "Help," said the flight agent. "Talk to her. What is her problem? We told her the flight was going to be late and she did this." I stooped to put my arm around the woman and spoke haltingly. "Shu-dow-a, Shu-bid-uck Habibti? Stani schway, Min fadlick, Shu-bit-se-wee?" The minute she heard words she knew, however poorly used, she stopped crying. She thought the flight had been cancelled entirely. She needed to be in El Paso for major medical treatment the next day. I said, "No, we're fine, you'll get there, just later, who is picking you up? Let's call him."

We called her son. I spoke with him in English. I told him I would stay with his mother until we got on the plane and ride next to her. She talked to him. Then we called her other sons just for the fun of it. Then we called my dad and he and she spoke for a while in Arabic and found out of course they had ten shared friends. Then I thought just for the heck of it why not call some Palestinian poets I know and let them chat with her? This all took up two hours. She was laughing a lot by then. Telling of her life, patting my knee, answering questions. She had pulled a sack of homemade mamool cookies—little powdered sugar crumbly mounds stuffed with dates and nuts—from her bag, and was offering them to all the women at the gate. To my amazement, not a single woman declined one. It was like a sacrament. The traveler from Argentina, the mom from California, the lovely woman from Laredo—we were all covered with the same powdered sugar. And smiling. There is no better cookie.

And then the airline broke out free apple juice from huge coolers and two little girls from our flight ran around serving it and they were covered with powdered sugar, too. And I noticed my new best friend—by now we were holding hands—had a potted plant poking out of her bag, some medicinal thing, with green furry leaves. Such an old country tradition. Always carry a plant. Always stay rooted to somewhere. And I looked around that gate of late and weary ones and I thought, this is the world I want to live in. The shared world. Not a single person in that gate—once the crying of confusion stopped—seemed apprehensive about any other person. They took the cookies. I wanted to hug all those other women, too. This can still happen anywhere. Not everything is lost.[1]

## REFERENCES

Bauman, Z. (2003). *Liquid love*. Polity Press.

Cixous, H. (1991). *"Coming to Writing" and other essays* (S. Cornell, D. Jenson, A. Liddle, & S. Sellers, Trans.). (D. Jenson, Ed.). Harvard University Press.

de Waal, F. B. M. (2008). Putting the altruism back into altruism: The evolution of empathy. *Annual Review of Psychology*, 39, 279–300.

Jegatheesan, B. (2019). Influence of cultural and religious factors on attitudes toward animals. *Handbook on Animal-Assisted Therapy*. https://doi.org/10.1016/B978-0-12-815395-6.00004-3

Lane, K. (2014). *Life on the edge*. John Blake Publishing.

Løgstrup, K. E. (1997). *The ethical demand*. Notre Dame Press.

Merleau-Ponty, M. (1994). Eye and mind. In G. A. Johnson (Ed.), *The Merleau-Ponty aesthetics reader: Philosophy and painting* (pp. 121–64). Northwestern University Press.

Orwell, G. (1949). *1984*. Harcourt.

van Heijst, A. (2011). *Professional loving care*. Peeters Press.

van Nistelrooij, I. (2014). *Sacrifice. A care-ethical reappraisal of sacrifice and self-sacrifice*. Peeters Press.

Waldenfels, N. (2016). Responsive love. *Primerjalna književnost (Ljubljana), 39*(1), 15–29.

Welz, C. (2015). In-between subjectivity and alterity: Philosophy of dialogue and theology of love. In U. Schmiedel & J. M. Matarazzo (Eds.), *Dynamics of difference: Christianity and alterity—A Festschrift for Werner G. Jeanrond* (pp. 125–134). Bloomsbury T&T Clark.

## NOTE

1. https://poets.org/poem/gate-4

# CHAPTER 3

---

# AFFECTION AND DUTY

---

When we say, "I love you," we are saying, "I care for you." Love is a form of care. According to some, it is the most authoritative form of caring (Frankfurt, 2004). Care can be enhanced by love, and both infuse the world with meaning. Care without love can be barren. Of course, they are not one and the same. Love can narrow care. Care can diminish love. At times they will be strange bedfellows. Often, they will sanctify each other.

To fail to care when one is called to care, is a failure of duty. It can also be a failure of hearing the call, or a failure to want to care. Care as duty is a hand that is multiply dealt. Whatever one's identity, that identity comes with responsibility, obligation, expectation. Also, our sense of self, of who we are, comes with desire. When persons care, they are willing to commit to their desire. They are not indifferent to the desire to care, they are prepared to act upon it, intervene, care. Our desire to sustain the care, however, can fade. Identity comes with opportunity to disappoint, to increase being hurtful, to diminish the care. Changing desires will change the care. Changing the care will change the duty, changing the duty will change the care.

A care ethic clings closely to the dealing out of duties. Any map of duties touches many regions of care. Not just *in extremis* but in ordinary hours of ordinary life, care of the spouse, care of the elder, care of the workmate, care changes. And thus, each caregiver is more deeply burdened, or relieved or replaced. Pairings, kinship, lending, borrowing, one relationship affects all the others. Caring is seldom a two-person game, for across

---

*a Paradigm of Care,* pp. 23–35

the table or soon at the door is another one loved or dependent or victim, needing attention, proposing alternatives, reworking the map of duty, of love, of desire and kinship.

How the folks respond, with or without conscious choice, changes the care, and even the care paradigm, the readiness to give care or be caring. Every smile, every wince counts. The affection, the duty. A care paradigm includes all the giving of care, but through understanding and expectation and reward, raises the opportunity for more care to be given.

But caring and caring to care can go wrong. Seeing the teacher as a critical caregiver, paleontologist and poet Loren Eiseley (1971) wrote, "the teacher is a sculptor of the intangible future. There is no more dangerous occupation on the planet, for what we perceive as our masterpiece may appear out of time to mock us—a horrible caricature of ourselves" (p. 200). Caring deeply has its risks. Caring can follow false pretenses. Caring can discourage the natural powers of recovery. Caring can misfit the need for respect. The perfect application of care lies beyond human attainment.

## DUTY

Duty is a human condition of obedience to a higher power. It needs not be, in fact it seldom is, in the modern West, a supernatural power. It is a circumstance felt by all people, more or less, and at most times, more at the back of their minds than the front. If we can believe our main sources of information:—TV news and Netflix serials, the dinner table, social media—duty is not much talked about. And yet we are propelled and restrained by a pretty strong sense of it. The confidences we hold, the liberties we take, the assessments we make of the casts within our contemporary life-dramas, are shaped by social pressure of such magnitude that that stuff can be considered our daily duty. We live up to it, whatever the higher power.

How is duty different from habit, persuasion, routine, and life-style? We think of it as a difference between choice and obligation. Care ethicists Inge Van Nistelrooij and Merel Visse (2019) wrote about the caregiver:

> Yet this practitioner also has the freedom to make moral decisions, to answer to or ignore moral appeals. Responsibility still appears as a moral task, as something one has or has not, and can decide about. This thought fits perfectly with the idea that freedom is required for morality, for without freedom (e.g., when coerced) one cannot be held responsible. But it also acknowledges givenness: that the caregiver is called upon, that a need is there that needs to be responded to. (Nistelrooij & Visse, 2019, p. 277)

Sometimes we follow a moral code, out of ethical persuasion, other times because we feel we are called upon. A fear of embarrassment of being exposed plays a part. We choose to be good, or bad, and we fear being caught out of line with "our guys." It is a mixed fuel that burns in our consciences.

Duty is associated with responsibility. Here, responsibility is literally a "having to respond." Not as in someone who makes a choice to respond to a hearing or seeing of a higher power, but as someone who has been given something that could not be heard or seen: a phenomenon that stirs something in us. It is as if we feel humbled by something that comes on our path as a sort of "gift," but that, at first instance, was not visible nor audible. Someone. Something. Or some event that makes us responsible without us even being aware of it, and without us wanting it. It is given to us involuntarily. Here, someone:

> at this moment, is not preceded by any vision or reason. Rather, the gifted "suffers from having to respond in the face of the phenomenon," and this suffering consists in the opening of a space that has been unforeseen and unimagined and is therefore filled with fright. Here opens a space of indecision that cannot be imagined without fright: the decision in favour of staging the given as a phenomenon, therefore also that in favour of the reason of things, can be made only without vision or reason since it makes them possible. (Nistelrooij & Visse, 2019, p. 280)[1]

Some work is in situations where behavior and violation are well spelled out and penalties are in view. Often the violations are more clearly defined, in a code or set of commandments, in generalities, more than in the specifics of the duty. Military service, jury duty, nursing, pharmacy, music, and sports all have codes of behavior that lead to punishment for violation of duty. The obligation is strong.

And yet duty is closely associated with the commitments of care, with mothering, with pastoral support, with veterinary specializations. Choices and obligations are mixed. The policing can be heavy or light. When it works, it works more because there is love, love of the ethic, of the profession, of the beneficiaries, whether prize-winning babies or horses gone lame. The line between love and duty lies behind a mist of human complexity.

## LOVE

The instances of personal care, in contrast to professional care, are frequently part of a loving relationship: spouses, parents and children, friends. Not all love is the same, as participants know. Each of us has a definition of each love, probably several. Love as an attitude, love as an emotion, a passion, love as relation with a beloved or a neighbor. Definitions, experiences, illustrations, memorabilia are all bound to cultures, religions, countries. We will not try to change your mind. But we cannot resist the urge to look closer at love's plurality, and at some of the contrasts. Love has been studied, categorized, celebrated, and blamed. Love can isolate, discriminate, lessening the disposition to care for others. The mixed message is found in this quotation from mystic Wahiduddin (Khan, n.d.):

> When we look at [it] from a mystic's point of view, we see that love has two aspects. Love in itself, and the shadow of love fallen on the earth. The former is heavenly, the latter is earthly. The former develops self-abnegation. In a person, the latter makes him more selfish than he was before. Virtues such as tolerance, mercy, forgiveness and compassion rise of themselves in the heart which is awakened to love.

Divine and human love need not be understood in opposition. Many of us know how closely these can be connected by our sensory organs. They are also connected with our vulnerability. Just take this brief description:

> It is raining outside; it is still warm, but it is raining—I see it through the window. The dog doesn't notice and is resolutely determined to go outside. Once downstairs, I notice that I have forgotten the umbrella. At first the rain is cool on my skin. It has immediately soaked my T-shirt. It strikes me coolly and then collects on my body in a layer of moisture. I endure it, standing in the rain for a moment and then slowly walking with my dog, who is without clothes and will be drenched (...) I accept it like an animal that belongs totally and completely to the world and is not separated from it, and suddenly I am filled with such joy and pleasure—in that moment I know that nothing bad can happen anymore. (Weber, 2014, p. 101)

By describing how he walks his dog in the rain, Andrew Weber, a German biologist, addresses his sense of aliveness, of being part of the world, of being connected to something bigger than himself. The world can be experienced as a *poetics of aliveness*, he argues. Him, putting himself and his dog in the streaming rain, produces meaning, it produces a love for the world, a care for rain, and desire for feeling the rain on his skin. At the same time, this happiness also bears a shadow, because it remains only for a while, then changes to something else, but there is always something that cannot be revealed or accessed. Our love and care for someone is always at the same time a separation. The mystics knew this. They also knew that we should not want to resolve this separation by trying to control it, because then the bond will not be alive. Uncertainty is the "necessary precondition for our ability to establish bonds with other beings" (Khan, n.d., p. 103). To care is to be alive within this situation of uncertainty. To be alive is to surrender to uncertainty and love. That requires courage because it alters things irrevocably.

Love and care are not necessarily bound to value. The care companion may be oh so dear to the other, but we do not necessarily care *because* we recognize his or her value. What I care about, or whom I love, acquires value just because I care about him or her. Here, care is a concern. Care can be seen as a disinterested concern for the existence of what/who we care for. We have the desire that the person or being or thing is not harmed. "Someone might care about social justice only because it reduces the likelihood of rioting; and someone might care about the health of another person just because she cannot be useful to him unless she is in good shape" (Frankfurt, 2004, p. 42).

Love is also an embrace; it is to be touched. Embrace as a sign of affection, of holding another in one's arms. Embrace comes from the old Latin *bracchium*, which means "arm." This bodily approach to love is about encircling, surrounding, enclosing someone. When we care, we put our arm around those who are in pain, showing compassion. Being embraced can bring us back to reality, it grounds us and stimulates physiological processes that slow down our nervous system, calming us. Being embraced and embracing someone makes visible the nature of who we are: relational beings, made of flesh and blood, with a need to be touched by others.

The mother who holds a child while breastfeeding, "holds" the child, surrounds it, protects it, and cares for it. Depriving a child of human touch can lead to lasting, lifelong damage. The embrace, the touch, is an emotional act for which meaning cannot be underestimated. This sheds a different light on the impact of social distancing in pandemic times, and on the separation of immigrant families at the U.S. border with Mexico. These children can suffer not being held or touched, which can lead to severe mental, emotional, and physiological problems. Colleen Kraft, President of the American Academy of Pediatrics, said:

> Their depression symptoms are just like adults. They stop eating, they stop sleeping ... I would be very concerned about children who have been on the border since April (...) These kids are going to be clamoring, crying for touch, and they're not getting it. (Roman, 2018, para. 13)

## THE ONE AND THE MANY

The caregiver works alone and with the many. A paradigm belongs to both, the one and the multitude. The caregiver may see but one beneficiary at a time but sees that person in the vast company of others cared for. The caregiver may see but one beneficiary at a time, but that beneficiary is also in the eyes and under the umbrella of all the caregivers of the world. The singular and the compound are orientations ever together. The care paradigm covers all.

> Tomas stays at home most of the time taking care of Marie who has dementia. Not a big problem, he's retired and can live on a modest pension. The children assure themselves he doesn't need their help quite yet, but they care, and in frequent ways, support care. Friends, those still around, care too, and show their kindness.

There is a history, multiple histories, a history of family life, another of work, of recovery from distress, histories of church and social security and safety protections. A population of caregivers has come together to build a society where the elderly and those with disability live in safety. Still the steps have their tumbles, and the meds do not always do their bidding. Tomas reflects on the comingling of helping hands.

> Marie is not sure who Tomas is, but it's good when he's with her. She keeps wanting "to go home," hoping her Mother would come get her. "What was that room with nurses? Is this a … can't think the name … a diaper? Seems a lot of grammas here. Yes, I'll hold the door."

> "What do you mean, Family Services is suffering a fourth consecutive loss? It's not supposed to make money. We pay taxes for those who need it. It doesn't matter what the newspaper says. It shouldn't be privatized. We care about those who can't afford Windsor Place." Tomas can't take care of Marie indefinitely.

Think of it this way. Everyone around cares about Marie. Not just her friends. Not just the people who moved here forty years ago. What is a care ethic if it is not a blanket for everyone? Even if you are poor, and you do not talk *esoterica*, and think the world has gone to hell, you care about people who are hurting, and wish there were a way that people would be taken care of—you are part of the *paradigm*. Care belongs to the many just as much as to the individuals. Each individual cares for lots of things, and each demographic superset of people cares for them too.

## AFFECTION AND TRUST

Let us not make too little of affection. If our children will in time take care of us only if they love us, let it so be. Even if we are skeptical of the deference and see it not as a duty but, at best, as a kind of fondness of decrepitude, let us accept the blessing. Just as we may have wondered if the gifts were truly a kindness, and not just a trade for affection or transportation, we should doubt that we can tell the true motive for the caring. Fake affection is far more common on the screen than in the living room.

Actually, suspension of suspicion is fundamental to good caregiving, just as to love. It is more common to speak of it as trust. Trust nourishes care. It is not a secret that care is given more readily when the giver is trusted to work in the best interests of the beneficiary. And not a secret that care is received more readily when the beneficiary is trusted to use the gift as intended. Alas, trust is not always deserved. Caregiving works among rich and poor, and in either sector there will be some caregivers who are intent on making the recipients poorer. It behooves those of us promoting a *care paradigm* to help with scam detection.

Pascal Collard and others (forthcoming) have scrutinized the role of trust in public policy and found no magic potion to enable trust. Trust remains a risky engagement, he argued. Certain conditions contribute to trust, however, such as honesty, tolerance in the community and loyalty to fellow community members.

## MARRIAGE

The universal concord of care and love is the marriage, not only the ceremony but the very life spent together. It is expected widely that the married couple will live under one roof, raise a family, share work, and care for each other with great regard in ordinary and extraordinary times. Much is offered in care, much is drawn from it. The giving and taking are themselves acts of love, sacrifice, cherishing, especially when the pain is almost too much to bear.

One version of Hindu wedding vows is as follows:

> With the first step, we will provide for and support each other.
> With the second step, we will develop mental, physical, and spiritual strength.
> With the third step, we will share the worldly possessions.
> With the fourth step, we will acquire knowledge, happiness, and peace.
> With the fifth step, we will raise strong and virtuous children.
> With the sixth step, we will enjoy the fruits of all seasons.
> With the seventh step, we will always remain friends and cherish each other.

Children grow up with the knowledge of marriage, that of their own parents and others close by. In their world of fictions, they see everlasting replays, joys and breakdowns, dependencies, and withdrawals. They find much for aversion, but later in their marriageable years they contemplate the rich rewards of care and love.

Stereotypes abound, but each vision of marriage is unique, born of personal experience, orchestrated by one's own family life in the special circumstances of each home. Much seems a given script, where choices are limited and predictable. And yet most hold the closest-known marriage as unique. And so, it is to be expected that standardized sustenance and remedy will not be good enough. The marriage counselor knows this, most mothers-in-law as well. A care paradigm is an infinite cabinet of applications, from Band-Aids to motorized wheelchairs, and an almost infinite cadre of rescuers and healers. Some of the best times of marriage are when spirits finally turn for the better.

## A Case of Marriage Counseling*

Thomas A. Seals, Jr.

*This case was used as a consultation specimen for individual professional review by 16 marriage counselors in Seals' dissertation research (Seals, 1985).

Lisa and Pete have been married about two years at the time of the video session. Lisa is about 25 years old, a woman of average height and weight. She has short, dark, curly hair, a pale complexion, and a roundish, pleasant, but tense face. She is dressed in jeans, a tweedy sports jacket, and loafers, casual, yet careful. Pete is in his early 30s. He is around six feet tall and on the lean side. His facial features are dominated by a moderately long, untrimmed beard and medium long brown hair. A ready, but somewhat forced, smile and eyes which seem to express pain are Pete's most visible features. He is dressed in jeans, a flannel shirt, and hiking boots, affecting a generally easygoing, "north woods" appearance.

The primary reason they give for coming into marital therapy is that they frequently get into "a kind of interaction where Lisa wants to get a response, and the more she probes, the less is there." Especially when Lisa is angry about Pete's lack of response, he freezes up and reports only feeling numb. Lisa alternatively gets more and more angry or withdraws into a discouraged silence.

This pattern of interaction seems especially distressing to Lisa because of the change it represents from their courtship. They met at their common workplace where both had responsible professional jobs in a research organization; Lisa was also pursuing an advanced degree. When they were first meeting and dating, Pete was very anxious to express his feelings to her and there had been plenty to express. He was married to Alice, which relationship he describes as being "a distant and cold" one. He had pursued Lisa vigorously while she was attempting to resolve a long term living together relationship with Martin, a man whose brilliance she nurtured and whose social incompetence she compensated for. Pete's attentions had been very flattering to her. She felt affirmed by Pete's interest in herself as a woman with intelligence and abilities and by his need for her nurturing and giving capacities.

For Pete, the change seems to be distressing mostly because it is distressing to Lisa. He has returned to a more normal way of being for himself after the painful experience of his divorce from Alice, intermingled with the excitement and anxiety associated with his quest for Lisa. Since both former relationships ended and they married, Pete has seemed most concerned about the extent to which he is acting toward Lisa and responding internally as his father did during Pete's years at home and even now. Lisa is also distressed at the prospect of Pete becoming more like his father, whom she "doesn't care for very much." She is especially worried about Pete's being a similar kind of father should they have children, a decision which they have been considering but choosing not to do yet.

They gave a couple of examples of how things seem to go amiss in their efforts to share or communicate intimacy with each other. A backdoor neighbor died, leaving an elderly widow. Initially, Lisa befriended her and visited regularly. Soon Pete joined her, and their visits with Agnes became almost a daily shared activity. When Lisa returned to school, Pete gradually seemed to take over their visits. He thought he was helping Lisa deal with a scarce time resource; she felt edged out of an important role and shared activity with Pete.

Second, Pete describes himself as being quite interested in domestic activities, especially cooking. He claims that he shows his caring for Lisa both by doing things for her, such as cooking and helping with her writing, and with hugs. He acknowledges some frustration at not being able to tell her what he is feeling for her. Lisa finds his ways of showing intimacy leaving her feeling not special and even abandoned emotionally. Her most prized attributes—being strong enough emotionally to be leaned on in a time of trouble, and being a loving and giving person, seem continually thwarted in their marriage by Pete's emotional withdrawal. She does not feel needed and feels that she gets a response from him only when she is herself in need of something from Pete. Both agree that their mutual decision-making "is the pits."

A good bit is said about their families. In addition to what has already been mentioned about Pete's father, he says that he is closer to his mother and that she always interpreted Pete's father's feelings to other family members. He remembers no open conflict between his parents at home. Only once, when he was 13 or 14, did he see his mother cry.

Considerably more attention is given to Lisa's family. Her father is described as a renowned scholar, busy, and demanding. Her mother seems to have been a woman of diverse and exceptional abilities. Lisa remembers her as one who "could do anything. She was a gourmet cook, she played the violin, she went back to work after 15 years of not working and made some really important contributions in what she was doing, published a lot of papers, and then she died." Lisa identifies herself as having worked partly through the grief over her mother's death, which occurred during Lisa's mid-teen years. The only time her more controlled and somewhat hard presentation during the session broke was when she was talking about her mother as the place from which love flowed in their family. She was teary and lost for words at that moment.

Lisa's mother could not, however, model achievement for her children without somehow diminishing their achievements by comparison. This surely seems to be the case with Lisa. Lisa always picked interests to develop which her mother did not have. She generally seems to take her achievements for granted, even deprecating them, as an expected result of being in a highly achievement-oriented family. She claims strongly to value her "nurturing and giving" qualities as what is special about her, not her accomplishments.

Of note in Pete's behavior in the session is the time when he was confronted by the woman therapist about the discrepancy between his smile and the painful experiences being discussed. A little later, he says, "It's scary, and I'm feeling a little disoriented right now. This whole routine about the smiling bit. I mean, that hit something inside me and I'm not all there right now."

## A PANDEMIC OF NEED FOR CARE

It does not serve our purpose here to think whether or not the need for care for Pete and Lisa is above or below average. Many individuals and couples with greater need have little access to marriage counseling. Pete and Lisa were in a situation where professional help was available, and they could afford it. But often it is not and the public should increasingly consider it necessary to provide it. But this book is not about care for people who need it and who recognize they need it and are in a position to get it. It is about opening spaces for people to care more, to work harder and reach further for a life space that helps people who have a need for help and do not understand the need and have little access to clarify the understanding and get the help.

Few readers will learn more about the pandemic of need for care by reading about Pete and Lisa. Most even recently have seen similar need on television, whatever channels are open. Many have read about it in commercial or social media. It could be they are less responsive because they see it so much, or because they are not in personal relationships with these people. Care, here, is devoted to helping others from a charitable concern, not because we love them personally, but as fellow humans and fellow custodians, the EMTs and CNAs of our world. Many people will reject the opportunity to respond to the need because the pandemic of care-need is so overwhelming, it is so incomprehensible, and it is so difficult to know where one's offering could actually be applied beneficially.

So, what is our duty? How do we change the world's disposition to help even a little? The need is so great and our leverage so small. First, it is important to acknowledge the obvious, that an armada of forces already exists. A D-Day intervention of landings, many of them referred to in this book. There are state and municipal programs, foundations, churches, professional associations, fraternities, and sisterhoods, and countless unions and collaboratives already committed, in whole or in part, to the improvement of care. The American Association for Adult and Continuing Education LEARNING EXCHANGE website includes information about their 2017 *Compendium* and other recent publications. For some, a place to start. But going further:

How do we change the world's disposition to help even a little? How could any response be effective? But changing the disposition, changing the awareness of bits that can be done, changing the commitment because the commitment is part of the good life, is reason enough to turn that way.

Although the leverage is small, the energy to apply to the levers to change the world is close at hand. The energy is close enough to touch. In every family, in every friendship, in every application for new work or new opportunity, one can scrape up an extra liminal of energy. The affection and sense of calling in every human relationship is there to be drawn upon. Almost every partnering contains more caring, available caring, than is being tapped. The reservoir is far from dry.

Advertising has taught us to be skeptical of merit, of scams, of miracles. We have to read the miraculous in our own hearts, and then to extend it further than our kith and kin, toward further needs than those already having professional attention, further than charity. We should not lessen our charities but should be ingenious in helping grow their reach.

How to do it? We do not know. Learn from Doctors Without Borders? Food Banks and Legal Aid Services have their start. There is a blanket of compassionate help around the world. But much too little. Should we not turn to those needs more than to fighting evils, evils like terrorists, drug traffickers, gun clubs, cults, enterprise zones? Should we withhold help because so many missions and crusades go wrong? Those answers belong to the implementation stage. Our job, dear reader, is to work on the understanding that the idea of a paradigm of care needs a much bigger embrace, extending to the very end.

### Caring for the Love of Your Life

Charles Cowger (2019)

Caregiving must be learned
crafted
has a costly tuition
is agile
depressing
savvy
sneaky
loving
a redefinition
It is more than a skill of coping
hoping
and when that fails
doping
It is not
hanging on to
what you've got
for dear life
no matter what …
what you've got
is not
Rather, it is about knowing new things about life
and being able to proceed
as if
they were true
Caregiving is what you do
with what
comes to you
when you have no clue
Few people seek it
nor wish to be good at it
something so vital
in finding out
what life is about
It makes some things more firm
some not
life as we had never learned

life as some will never understand
their loss
until they get their turn


## REFERENCES

Collard, P., Visse, M., Tonkens, E., & Leget, C. (forthcoming). *Enabling trust in collaborative social policy making: A literature review.*

Eiseley, L. C. (1971). The mind as nature. In *Night Country* (pp. 195–226). Scribner.

Frankfurt, H. (2004). *The reasons of love.* Princeton University Press.

Khan, H. I. (n.d.). *The spiritual message of Hazrat Inayat Khan.* Wahiduddin's web. https://wahiduddin.net/mv2/XI/XI_III_11.htm

Roman, C. (2018). *The lasting damage of depriving a child of human touch.* The Cut. https://www.thecut.com/2018/06/the-lasting-damage-of-depriving-a-child-of-human-touch.html

Seals, T. A., Jr. (1985). *A theoretical construction of gender issues in marital counseling.* (Doctoral dissertation), University of Illinois, College of Education.

Van Nistelrooij, I., & Visse, M. (2019). Me? The invisible call of responsibility and its call for care ethics: A phenomenological view. *Medicine, Health Care, Philosophy, 22,* 277.

Weber, A. (2014). *Matter and Desire: An Erotic Ecology.* White River Junction, VT: Chelsea Green Publishing.

## NOTE

1. The quote has been slightly adjusted. In addition: "the subject is not in the nominative case, nor in the accusative. Rather, the subject is in the dative: he or she is "the gifted," that Is, the "unto whom/which" or the one to whom has been given."

# CHAPTER 4

---

# MORALITY AND RELIGION

---

Two young hitchhikers were about to squeeze into the back seat of the VW Bug, when a burly Rabbi yanked them aside and crawled in himself. He looked weary, probably having prayed at the Wailing Wall all day. What does religion have to do with morality?

To the driver, a fellow resident of Jerusalem, this Rabbi seemed called by a strange God. Surely he had been worshipping, praying, since early sun. "Oh, the depth of the riches and wisdom and knowledge of God. How unsearchable are his judgments and how inscrutable his ways!"[1] And the ways of a Rabbi. The ways of Aggressors are many. And the ways of Caring are many.

> When the imam gave the word, the Muslims bowed with their hands crossed over their bodies, then dropped to their knees and pressed their heads to the ground. A woman with a toddler sheltered her child beneath her body. The woman in her wheelchair tipped as far forward as she could without falling out. When everyone repeated the movement a moment later, it was like watching a huge, perfect wave curl and fall with a rush toward the shore. (Taylor, 2019, p. 128)

The stones of our mosques and churches are manifestation of our caring. They belong to that dominion of caring that celebrates communion, that works to bring holy and heathen to the alter, and together to a place of reconciliation. The temples place faith in hierarchy, to a higher being and

---

a shared discipline. There is rank and file, but also gospel singing and pastoral care.

If we were to have had a meter rating the popularity of religion around the world, we think we would have seen a tumble and spill. People shudder at terrorists in spiritual rage, pedophilia, social action working from church basements, vacant pews. Not all news has been bad. Cults are diminishing, the Pope and Dalai Lama are progressive, once again no one objects to prayer in those schools still doing it, megachurches have full parking lots, the National Football League (when operating) tries not to start games before coffee in Fellowship Hall. Still, in many parishes, *pro-life* is the activist voice of morality.

But that that is aggregated, distilled, across nation and world as a whole, is not as important as what happens, in each home and shelter and penthouse and sampan, that which is experienced as good and caring by individual persons. Tallies on checklists are one of the signs of amorality, not morality. The standards of a caring world are set, need be set, in each person's every experience. It is set on what is right in the situation. And what is right in the hearts and minds of individuals. One against one against one is not necessarily chaos. It could be humanist heaven.

Righteousness is not found in a book, or produced from a mosque, or distilled from a voting booth, or deconstructed from situation comedies. Righteousness is a human commodity, molded by the movement and judgment of all the people, individually and in relationships, and little found in tallies and metersticks. Righteousness could exist in any form, in cellular form, yet also in any aggregate of cells. It is not available to sensory experience but is intuitively known and spiritually felt. Righteousness is sampled on cell phones, in the exhaustion of work, in sighs and hugs, in matters of conscience.

Goodness and evil are but one blanket, covering all that we do; one warmth and chill, penetrating, radiating, all that we are. Warmth and chill fill empty spaces as well as the occupied, knowing no bounds. Yet they are nothing without the human knowing of them. They have no domain of their own, for they are conceived by and nurtured and cared for and terminated by the creatures who share language and thought. When they leave that awareness, goodness and evil cease to exist.

## HUMAN EXPERIENCE

Awareness is not a matter of definition or sensory registration. It is a matter of knowing, of interpreting, of connecting the human experiences. Those experiences can be registered in many ways, particularly by artists and editors and children's choirs, but it is borne by individual experience.

All knowledge shares the same carrier, fired by the same propellant. Albert Einstein was said to have said, "All evidence is the evidence of human experience."

Human experience seems a deep ocean, but human populations have not been huge for long. Blogwriter "eukaryote" wrote in his/her "Funnel of Human Experience" (eukaryote, 2018) that "half of human experience has happened after 1309 A.D.," and that "15% of all experience has been experienced by people who are alive right now." Whether he has got it exactly to the year is not the point. Very little else has happened because there has been almost no-one here until now.

To be sure, religious experience, worship, wonder, has had a considerable history, but if experience were taken as the sum total and not the calendar of human experiencing, then we today are directly in touch with much of the sum total, and adding second-hand experience, we have much more. It is the difference in cultures rather than the difference in centuries that gives experience its color and variety. And thus too, the spiritual side of caring will reflect the diversity of its contexts, the contexts we have tried to think about in this book.

> Tomas and Marie had wanted their children to have religious education, so took them to Sunday School. But when the kids got older, they refused to go to church. They said, "There might have been miracles back then, but not anymore." Marie told them that spirituality was more a matter of caring than of having miracles.

Caring is morality, a prism of righteousness, and part of spirituality. Caring is responding to the call, hearing the needs of another, fulfilling our promises. A paradigm of care embraces not so much the acts of caring, essential though those be, but embraces the grand expectation of caring and being cared for. The paradigm is a caring ethic. Our agents, our caregivers, our worldly angels, make it possible for us to know the care ethic, whether or not we share the joy and despair of the beneficiaries. They are mothers and fathers, daughters and sons. They, those care-givers, are also the priests, pastors, monks and nuns, imams, sensei, ministers, and bishops of human care.

Just to be human is to be a caregiver. Caregivers weave the social net. Some do it not so well. Many do it well, even as if genetic divination. Most do it with too little reward. Many do it without awareness that their attitudes and their comfort are the buoyancy and sweetness of the situation. Let us say it again and again, a care paradigm is devotion and salvation compounded of the human essences of every saint and sinner. Here words from Lauren Eiseley (1971, p. 176):

And yet, plunged as I am in dire memories and midnight reading, I have said that it is the sufferer from insomnia who knits the torn edges of men's dreams together in the hour before dawn. It is he who from this hidden, winter vantage point sees the desperate high-hearted bird fly through the doorway of the grand hotel while the sleepy doorman nods, a deed equivalent in human terms to that of some starving wretch evading Peter at heaven's gate, and an act, I think, very likely to be forgiven.

It is a night more mystical however, that haunts my memory. Around me I see again the parchment of old books and remember how, on one rare evening, I sat in the shadows while a firefly flew from volume to volume lighting its small flame, as if in literate curiosity. Choosing the last title it had illuminated, I came immediately upon these words from St. Paul: "Beareth all things, believeth all things, hopeth all things, endureth all things." In this final episode I shall ask you to bear with me and also to believe.

Our friend, hospice worker Terry Denny said, "I ask them two questions. Do they want me there? And do they want me to talk? The rest works out however it can." Terry wrote a book, *Being with the Dying* (Denny, 2016). One of his stories was the following:

## Leslie, Charles and I: A Hospice Volunteer's Confession

Terry Denny, *University of Illinois*

Because my visits as a Hospice volunteer with Leslie lasted five months, I had a wonderful opportunity to observe, reflect, learn, and try to be helpful.

At the top of over a hundred small pages of notes, written after my visits with Leslie in her condo, I often scribbled "Another LL" (Leslie Lesson). I am a tournament-level note taker.

I come to see life as a long series of lessons. During my early and middle adult years, I saw myself as a competent teacher—an achiever if you will. But now, as a Hospice volunteer in my 70's, I'm viewing things quite differently—especially after being with Leslie and Charles, who conducted a workshop *On Dying* for the Medical Center Hospice Program during the period that I was with Leslie.

Charles' workshop left me with itches I was unable to scratch—and Leslie didn't respond in the way I expected—although I'd already been with several patients who had died. In fact, I had become satisfied with my competence as a volunteer Hospice worker. My self-assurance would be challenged by my weeks with Leslie.

My early notes included, "Is she keeping me at arms' length? What am I doing wrong?" At first, I suspected that the *distance* I felt in our relationship had something to do with my being a man. She was, after all, my first female Hospice patient, and, honestly, I felt a little unsure of myself.

Six months later, I was even less sure of myself—but it had little to do with my being a man. In retrospect, I had missed an important clue in our first meeting when Leslie greeted me at her door saying, "Things have certainly been busy lately." I should have listened and picked up on her lead, but didn't. My notes about that visit were sparse. I had missed the significance of her feeling "busy."

I called early in the next week to make an appointment for a second visit—only to hear her say, 'No, don't come. I feel a little tired this week." Fair enough. I called three days later and we set a new date and time.

Notes indicate we spent a "splendid afternoon together" during that visit. We "traded stories about our first dates, first childhood romance, first cars." Now we were getting somewhere, I thought! I could hardly wait for next week.

Alas, she called to cancel: "Just not feeling up to it." That bruised my ego. What am I doing wrong? What should I change in my approach? Am I being too candid? Am I asking the wrong questions? Perhaps I look or behave like someone she dislikes? What is going on here?

I called our coordinator of volunteer workers, who assured me that she would check into it. Her return call comforted me when she said that Leslie was, "OK with me." She also suggested that I talk with Jerome.

Jerome, the Hospice social worker for Leslie's case, startled me by suggesting that Leslie probably had more important things on her mind than me. That wasn't very comforting.

By now, the reader should be thinking, "Terry's narrative seems to be pretty much about the palliative care of *himself* rather than of Leslie the patient.

During my fourth visit, Leslie let me in on a profound secret when she said, "I suppose you know this already, but dying requires a lot of thought.

In truth, I had not.

Leslie went on, "Dying takes a lot of thought and concentration—all of you, your whole self." There was a long silence.

"It's not only the problem of having this illness. I need more time *alone* than what I am now getting."

For the first time I heard and understood. She needs time, alone.

So, I spoke with the daytime home aide about Leslie taking walks, reading her book outside, creating time to honor her need for privacy. I noted it in my Hospice report as well.

Marking time. My next few visits seemed to go OK. We visited two or three times a week. I had learned from earlier patients that, if the patient is up to it, doing something purposeful together could be a good thing. I kept listening for Leslie to suggest what that might be.

One day she said, "I could use some help with a stack of mail." That afternoon we shredded the unwanted mail that had been piling up for a month or so. Shredding proved to be a purposeful activity that prompted conversation about life, values, and what lay ahead.

Leslie loved to shred. She would pick up an envelope, read it, offer a social commentary about a charitable organization, or a correspondent, or a sales pitch within a mass mailing. "I'm not a cheapskate—but I 'm not a fool either. How many times a year do they have these fund drives?"

"You contribute to this one, don't you?" [American Cancer Society]? "You should," she exclaimed.

Another piece of mail elicited, "American Airline—AA Literature." [Her husband was an American pilot.] "Flying; oh, so much fun. Flying is more than getting from one place to another. It's about freedom. Well, it was about freedom. Nowadays there's way too much time spent on the tarmac to feel free." Freedom, independence and control proved to be recurrent themes for Leslie.

Watching television hardly qualifies as purposeful activity for me, but it proved to be so throughout the middle months of my journey with Leslie. We watched televised golf matches, which prompted her to make several sage observations about the nature of the sport and what it had meant to her.

"When I played golf, I always tried to respect the game and the people I played with. For me, there are far too many people on the course who are playing at golf, playing around on the course, not playing the game as it was meant to be played. They make 'mulligans,' pick up short putts and improve their lie without regard for the game."

In her estimation she was not a very good golfer, but declared, "I was always the best person I could be on the course." A picture of a proud, independent, strong-willed woman was starting to emerge. I did a lot of listening.

During my next visit Leslie pointed to a small model of a Chevrolet convertible on the top of her TV. "Now there's the best car I ever had! I worked as a nurse during the Second World War. I bought that car with my money.

"Remember I worked twelve hours for seven dollars. No way to get rich. But, there's something to be said for a woman owning her own car and I did. Cost me $800. My Chevy Deluxe convertible was the cat's meow in squadron gray with red leather trim. I sold it a year later for $750 and bought a sheared beaver fur coat. What do you think of that? I bought our marriage license with my own money. Remember, it was wartime and women had to take care of things."

In the following weeks Leslie observed: "I have friends who are vacationing out here and want to visit. I almost want to say, 'I am not up to it. Please don't come.' But of course, I won't say that. My daughter is being so strong. She knows everything I want and need. I keep getting more than I need."

The director of a Hospice Program in San Francisco spent a day with Hospice volunteers and staff in his home. Charles addressed a fundamental issue in the workshop: Why is a Hospice volunteer with the patient? Charles warned us about volunteers having agendas. Did I have an agenda: Of course I did. I vowed to lessen it.

I was learning more and more about Leslie's earlier days—but little about her sense of dying. Her feelings and thoughts about dying came when out of the blue she said, "I never expected this time to be so boring. But I'm lucky not to be in much pain." Here was a chance to "bear witness." Here was a chance to be thoughtful about what was happening to Leslie and my reactions to it. Here was a chance to turn toward Leslie's and my suffering —but I couldn't and just sat there and said nothing.

"Good neighbors stop in unannounced. Old friends and family have come from afar. Well-wishers call me and old friends in the area come by. I don't need 24 hours-a-day coverage, but I've got it. All this Hospice care. I appreciate it but ... this is all too much; it just wears me out. Sometimes it seems like I almost have one performance after another...."

It is getting harder and harder for me to even stand. It's getting harder and harder to do everything. I am getting tired so easily. The body ... the body. Have you ever noticed how some people confuse physical incompetence with mental incompetence?"

"Yes," I thought, "I'm guilty." I was soon to learn even more about becoming a better Hospice volunteer.

After the workshop I sought clarity about my motives as a Hospice worker. I seemed to me that there was too much I and Me in my thinking and not enough of Leslie.

I tried to park my agenda before entering a conversation on the phone or being in person with Leslie. It sounded easy—but it was not easy for me. I have always seen myself as an action kind of guy. I have always worked hard to *fix* things as a husband, father, grandfather, professional educator. I found and continued to find it difficult to accept Charlie's message about how seeing and respecting the patient is more important than one's self view and action.

I thought I had been working hard on my listening skills with patients so I could do something. Charles did not agree with that goal. He advised that it required a kind of discipline of self to make room for the other person. It turns out that what I wanted to do is far less important than sensing what the patient is thinking and feeling.

Charles deeply disturbed me and I don't like to be disturbed. The kind of compassion that Charles and Leslie were calling for required me to be aware profoundly of the patient's suffering.

Simone Weil, in *Waiting for God*, writes, "We don't want to contemplate it [allowing suffering to disturb us]. However, those who suffer have no need for anything in this world but for people capable of giving them attention. The capacity of giving one's attention to a sufferer is a very rare and difficult thing. It is almost a miracle: it is a miracle."

A new start? On my way to my next meeting with Leslie (after Charles' workshop), I impetuously bought a bouquet.

Our team's social worker told me that Leslie had not been taking her depression medication and was feeling low. I finally understood that Leslie was tired of being visited and didn't need a visitor just because he wanted to visit.

I learned to accept that much of what I had been doing wasn't right because it wasn't what Leslie needed. Entering Leslie's room with an orchid plant, I recall mumbling something about her might liking some spring posies. She smelled the plant, inspected each bloom and chirped, "I'm so happy you brought these."

She went on to tell me about her diminished vision due to macular degeneration. The possibility of blindness struck more fear in her heart than did her imminent death. Her wit often calmed my troubled heart—especially about such large matters. Leslie said, "I sure hope this [cancer] plays out in the right order; first you die, then you can't see."

She stared outside, cried softly for a minute or so and proclaimed she was certainly lucky not to be in pain. Charles shared his view of empathy, which he felt Hospice volunteers need in their work. "Empathy is moving about delicately in the patient's world without judgment." Leslie had invited me into her world. I sat—just being with her....

However alike and different, morality and religion are defined by human experience. The reciprocity of Terry and Leslie in their mutual respect, of honoring and of love, is not so much a matter of code and creed, but more a matter of care and caring. We will dig deeper into the experience of reciprocity in Chapter 6. For the moment, think of the awareness of each other, the matter of knowing, of interpreting, of connecting human experiences. To repeat, those experiences can be registered in many ways, particularly by artists and editors and children's choirs, but it is borne by individual experience as in the case of Terry and Leslie.

We can live our lives quietly. John Milton spoke of the quiet of his devotion in a poem repeated here toward the end of Chapter 10. He spoke in the language of poetry. He spoke. The character of devotion is realized in experience, but it exists in its human strength especially when it is expressed in language. The quality of caring can be quiet, but it often needs the complexity of expression. Our experience is enriched by the freedom we have to express the virtues of morality and religion.

## FREEDOM OF EXPRESSION

The First Amendment to the U.S. Constitution states:

> Congress shall make no law respecting an establishment of religion, or prohibiting the free exercise thereof; or abridging the freedom of speech, or of the press; or t he right of the people peaceably to assemble, and to petition the Government for a redress of grievances.

Although this prohibition is placed on the U.S. Congress, it is taken to mean a protection of the rights of each individual citizen: a freedom of religion, of speech, and of assembly. That is, a protection against restraint by the authorities and other citizens. It grants freedom of expression.

The authors of the Bill of Rights were prescient and far-sighted in seeing needs for these protections, but they were near-sighted about some others. They did not include social press and misinformation as similar threats to equanimity. They did not adequately calculate the intrusiveness and injury of bullying and stereotyping and racial discrimination. They did not adequately calculate the distortion and compulsion of advertising and misinformation campaigns, the disquiet and hurt, and thus, the need for care.

The general public is quite able to rationalize for itself some of the unrelieved social conditions, but the people become even less responsive to cries for help when the problem is poorly understood by community members. For years, a newspaper columnist attacked the unprofitability of the municipal home for the elderly, until the citizens no longer saw it as a public asset. Federal spokespersons treated reports of politically embarrassing conditions as needing the confidentiality of national security classification. The Russian government accused the Ukrainian government of interfering with the 2016 U.S. elections when, by mass digital repetition, they had themselves done the interfering.

Whether oral or written, our social media messages, temporal, with few paper trails, leave little evidence of what happened or what was said, thus make misrepresentation commonplace. Advertising, whether oral or written, has itself no standard of honesty, no morality. The checks and balances of government so delicately framed in the Constitution have been found ineffectual. The contexts of contemporary living have great streams of deceit.

Deceit plays both ways. It is deceit to ask others about their health, when little cared about, although it regularly makes both of us feel better. It is deceit to send Christmas cards, although hardly worth a Hail Mary. It is a deceit to include source references in your research report, while showing your author friends you care about them, to enhance the appearance of your scholarship. Amazon has a trove of books about lying (e.g., Harris & Harris, 2013). Freedom of expression carried too far.

Peccadillos perhaps, but, in full force, they add up to an ethic running counter to the caring ethic. Good human relations rely on honesty, sincerity, trust. We enjoy metaphor, satire, absurdity but they push toward an expectation that all is in jest, all needing quibble, not to be taken seriously. We used to say in derision, innocence is bliss, but now we realize, it is true, that awareness, doubt, skepticism, and critique are doubly clouded, chasing bliss. When exposed, the infirmity of the world clouds our personal firmaments. We too need care. We need the assurance that others care. Others far and wide. We need greeting cards and email to express our needs for connection. For all its vices, internet does us good. It expands the artists' markets. More kids call home. It voices opportunity. Isn't there greater opportunity to be heard?

## THE GOLDEN RULE

Speaking of undercutting the verities, there is something wrong with the Golden Rule. Do unto others as you would have them do unto you. Unless you think about it, it seems a pretty good way to be a caregiver. The Golden Rule is pretty popular among us do-gooders around the world. According to Wikipedia ("Golden Rule," n.d.):

> "the idea dates at least to the early Confucian times (551–479 BC)," and appears "prominently in Buddhism, Christianity, Hinduism, Judaism, Taoism, Zoroastrianism, and "the rest of the world's major religions." 143 leaders of the world's major faiths endorsed the Golden Rule as part of the 1993 "Declaration Toward a Global Ethic.... Simon Blackburn states that the Golden Rule can be "found in some form in almost every ethical tradition."

But it declares we should treat others as we would have them treat us. How many people in the world know how we ought to be treated? Do we really believe that our lives are so similar, that our needs so common, that our safety so well defined, that those folks should choose what is best for us? But disregard that. This is not a book on care-getting. This is a book on caring. One of its main points is that care needs to be put together in ways that fit the needs, the personalities, the situations of the individuals needing care.

For how many people in this world would the care that we would choose for ourselves be the right care for them. Some, but not enough for the Golden Rule to be a good standard of care for humankind. It should not be expected that in defining a care for a particular soul or sect that we should completely ignore how valuable it would be for ourselves. But the far more important definition is how to conceive of good care for that soul or sect *in its particular situation* as they see it. Do unto others as they themselves would have it done.

When we look at the famous painting by Norman Rockwell (see Figure 4.1), we see the near and the far of Bogardus social distance. We ask ourselves—however much or little we might like to be hugged by each of them—how many of them would like to be hugged by us? Or touched? Or married? Actually, the idea that humanity's standard should be set by our personal preferences is off toward outrageous.

To be a caring person, to promote the caring ethic, one needs to be able to figure out what is, for "others," a relief, a blessing, a respect, an act of love. Not easy. Of course, one reads the signs of response, the sigh, the smile, the words of gratitude. But we have to be aware that we will not always get an honest showing. Sometimes they are merely tolerating us caregivers, but ethically cannot express it. Clearly, we should not suppose

**Figure 4.1**

*The Golden Rule by Norman Rockwell*

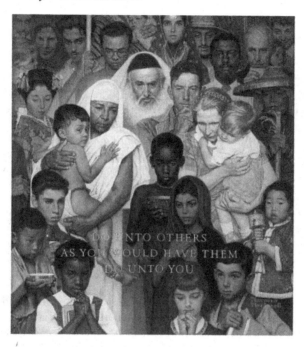

NORMAN ROCKWELL MUSEUM

that we know how we would feel were we in their place. We must try to know how our help is of value, but clearly, we dare not just do as we would have them do unto us.

All too often, neither those "others" know, nor do we know, what is the right thing to be one. Should they hear another story? Should they have a cookie? Should they be encouraged to talk about death and dying? We cannot know for sure. The care ethic is not easy to practice. But we can work to understand what those, for whom we give care, would welcome and what might be hurtful to them. Their request is first and foremost, but then there's more. Our view needs to be broad, as open as possible to not only hear, but to listen. We need to listen to hear the prices paid for our caregiving.

Each group of helpers itself needs care. Some institutions have managed to live a long life, devoted to giving care: for example, the Salvation Army. As Mrs. Pring says, "Keeping going is not easy." This interpretive report came from England at an earlier time, 1969.

## Saved by the Army

David Jenkins, 1969 (DRJ)

A report by Professor David Jenkins on the visit paid by Form 4B of
Bolthole Secondary Girls School to the Ethel Street Salvation Army
Hostel, as part of an evaluation of the University of Keele/Schools Council
Integrated Studies Project, directed by David Bolam. DRJ was invited
because of the relevance of this particular visit to the "Outgroups in
Society" pack material (Stenhouse, 1973, pp. 305–321).

The coach left at 1 P.M., driven by one Brian Hudson who exerts an interesting influence on the team. Mary Brown: *I like the new pack (of learning
materials) enormously, and felt I could give it to Brian. He's Salvation Army, you
know. He's got contacts, you see.* Brian is in coach hire, is friendly and operates
at low rates. In discussing his choice, Brian suspects that he is motivated
by a desire to protect the girls from the seamy side of life. He positively
refused to arrange a visit to the Ramla Street Men's Hostel, possibly reflect-
ing an Army preference for the more PRO-conscious Ethel Street outfit.

The outward journey is jovial. The teachers and DRJ sit at the front.
Brian plays pop, medium-loud, on the coach radio. All admonition is done
by Brian. (*Sit down girls, or I'll stop the coach.*) The girls file out at the hostel
and are counted, in case any decide to stay.

The hostel itself is uncompromisingly depressing. A decrepit building in
a rundown and derelict slum area, it maintains an authentic "brands from
the burning" image, piety in the face of squalor. A board outside proclaims
in lamb-blood red that this is the "Rehabilitation" Centre of the Salvation
Army's Men's Social Services. The place is run by Captain Robert Pring and
Mrs Pring.

The physical organization of the building lends itself to an interpretation of three symbolic levels. Upstairs are the cubicles and bedrooms. We
are invited to tour these and view the cramped bunks with fleur-de-lys and
buckled-belt blankets, that must remind the inmates that these are SALVA-
TION ARMY and not personal possessions. Indeed, there is little evidence
anywhere of a personal signature (contrast student rooms in colleges) and
I wondered if in fact it was not untypical of the regime that the tour of the
charitable works involved what in other circumstances would be a clear
invasion of privacy.

The second symbolic level is the "middle earth," lying immediately
below the dubious heaven. This is taken-up by an enormous chapel and
a kitchen that services more temporary human needs. Above the table
and the pulpit is an enormous repulsive sentimental Christ (later referred
to colleague Mary as *that signed portrait of Jesus with eyes that follow you
everywhere*. Around the walls are the Olly choruses uneasily reminiscent of
my Welsh chapel days:

My sins are gone, gone, gone
Far far far away.

and incomprehensibly:

> Cheer up ye saints of God
> There is nothing to worry about (!)

This would possibly have offered some reassurance to the fragmentary personalities in care were it not for the symbolic ritual associated with the passage of time (ever a noncomformist preoccupation). The building is full of massive clocks, going quite beyond the questionable need to know the time in this twilight world. Each clock carries a card with the uncompromising message:

> Time gentlemen please!
> Time to turn to Christ.

This reference to the pub-culture is later to seem even stranger. Although DRJ did not see it himself, Mary later assured him that the actual numerals on one of these timepieces were replaced by the letters DECISION TIME.

Whether the "saints" in fact had anything "to worry about" was puzzlingly difficult to establish. One would be tempted to describe the descent to the lower sweathouse as a guided tour under the direction of Captain Guido de Montefeltro, but the metaphor would be lost on those either unfamiliar with Dante's *Inferno* or inhibited from using it in this context. The working conditions downstairs are incredibly cramped, squalid, and overcrowded, and it would be difficult to imagine them not in breach of the Factory Acts. The men work with anything from manic intensity to total disaffection. They sit cheek-by-jowl, elbow-to-elbow on "piecework" production of paper bags for a supermarket. Phrases from Tawney's *Religion and the Rise of Capitalism* flicker across the consciousness. There is a smell of unwholesomeness that one or two girls try to work back within their conventional understanding. *(Captain and Mrs Pring must be wonderful people to work and live in this smell.)*

The men themselves? They were clearly and visibly the flotsam and jetsam of our society, unkempt, shuffling, often with deranged or vacant expressions. Most had histories of mental illness or psychological breakdown. A number had come from Worrell Street Hospital under a questionable referral system. *(The doctor will ring up and say "Captain Pring, we have some that you could take.")* They are docile and friendly, and respond touchingly to the thin trail of pretty girls tripping innocently through their part of the human icefield. *(How is it then? Aye, Aye? Where do you come from, love? Is them students of yours?)* They had the kind of contentment that is born of resignation. *(Can't grumble. It's all right here; you know what I mean?).*

DRJ goes back to talk to James Burke. Jimmy has added just a little to that aching "hollowness within" that results from any contact with real human plight. He is not in the main workshop but DRJ catches sight of his hollow-eyed and stubbled face peering out of a coalhouse-like extension, and goes over to join him. What is his job?

*I peel potatoes. I don't work for "him up there" but work for the cook.* He complained without emphasis of the regime, glancing around carefully before continuing:

*They're religious fanatics, you know what I mean? I've been around you see. Different when you've been around. It's all right. I'm content, you know what I mean? It's good enough for such as me.*

He earns 10 shillings per week, but some of those on piecework are able to earn up to 30 shillings. This ceiling figure was later defended by the management as being due to some MSS benefit complications. On the surface it seems wrong for mental defectives to be on piecework in 19th-century factory conditions and picking up 30 shillings per week, but normal notions of dignity and responsibility may not apply. One wonders about the purely commercial aspects. (How much are the bags sold for? DRJ resolves to ask Mary Brown to find out.) Does the alleged dignity of manual (and profitable) labor rule out art therapy, for example?

Jimmy Burke described the institutional setting very much in a "management and men" framework. His "definition of the situation" contrasted quite remarkably with the official account. "The men" resent the "exploitation" and see themselves working for less than fair reward, but on the other hand they need the security and are unwilling to venture out. Apparently, in some of them, this lack of confidence is pathological, but in no sense is rehabilitation a firm goal of the management. This worried Ivan Richards more than anything else.

*(Oh, just one or two leave us,* explained Mrs Pring, *but that's usually when a cousin or somebody insists on taking them. It's stupid really, as they soon find out when they can't cope. The men get worse than ever and end up back in Worrell Street.)*

The impression that overwhelmed your observer, quite literally, could be summed up in the words "captive congregation."

Let Mr Burke continue his story. *He's not like us; him. up there,* confided Jim (he never referred to Captain Pring by name, let alone rank). *You know? He tells us we are working for the Lord.* (He looked down unbelievingly at the bucket of peeled potatoes.) *The men down here,* he confided, *ARE WORKING FOR THEIRSELVES.*

... And all this compulsory chapel, you know what I mean?

DRJ: Are you sure it's compulsory?

Jim (slyly): Well, they say you're expected to go. You know what I mean?

DRJ: You mean it's easier to go?

Jim: I mean you've got to go.

By the time your lurker rejoins the main group, the chapel houses all the Bolthole Girls, and Captain Pring is "putting them in the picture" about Army work in general. Mrs Pring stands near the door, but chips in when she feels a contribution would be useful. The effect is less of informality than a sort of tag-wrestling. Captain Pring is talking about the "For God's Sake Care" campaign (a brilliantly effective advertising-agency job) and drawing attention to the photograph of the pregnant thirteen-year-old whose condition (we were solemnly informed) *arose directly out of her own father's deed.* A phrase to savor. Captain Pring is an attractive personality, open and brisk. His wife is oddly paradoxical: warmly mothering and sharply narrow at one and the same time. They are both paternalistic in their attitude towards their duties.

*These are weak, childlike personalities.*
*We have to think for them.*

The girls ask a number of questions about the gift of shirts that the school had made, and obviously feel pleased that they had helped. DRJ very politely and tentatively asks if religious service is compulsory. Both answer immediately and together that it is optional, quite optional. *But we have a full house every Sunday. Everybody comes because they want to,* explained Mrs Pring. It was a helpful reply.

DRJ asks, again with care, whether fragmentary personalities may not actually be put under pressure by all the clocks and emphasis on the responsibility for repentance. *Is Salvationism in fact inappropriate in what must in some respects resemble a mental hospital?*

But apparently DRJ had got it wrong again. There is no pressure. They sing choruses. It is all warm and reassuring.

(Cheer up ye saints of God
There is nothing to worry about.)
*What are they, up there?* DRJ asks Jim, feigning ignorance.
*They're salvationists, you see; that's what they are, salvationists.*
DRJ: *What does that mean?*
*Well, not like Catholics. You know what I mean? They take all the bits of the Bible. You know what I mean? The bits about the blood. They're fanatics, you see. You know what I mean?*
(I think I know what he means.)

Later Mrs Pring bemoans the cramped premises. (Jim had previously told me that most of them crept over to the Cobblers Tavern for the odd evening drink.) She wishes that there were recreational facilities.

DRJ: *Aren't there any pubs around here that the men can go to?*

Mrs Pring treats the matter with contempt. *(Oh we discourage that kind of thing. Besides some of them are on tablets, and it wouldn't do if they saw the others going.)* When she talked of her vocation, actually living there on a pittance, one could excuse her General Booth-like attitude to the drink problem, itself "traditional." She is quite literally, in her eyes, surrendering her life to God. One felt genuinely sorry that so much of what we had seen, was for other reasons disturbing.

Eventually the farewells. In the coach on the way back, Ivan Richards draws attention good-humouredly to a seedy shop uncompromisingly labelled RICHARDS BANKRUPTCY BARGAINS. The laughter is polite, and the girls thoughtful.

Later Mary and I talked at the school gates to a group of girls. They said they felt "very depressed" but couldn't quite explain why. When we gave our comments, they acknowledged recognition, almost with surprise (*Yeah, that's just how I felt*). The disturbing element had been without a doubt the quality of the lives of the inmates. If these were the saved, they did not want to be taken to see the lost.

Ivan goes about some business and I talk to Mary in the staffroom. She is a very perceptive and interesting person. Her depression about it all expressed itself in symbolic anger at the big Jesus with the staring eyes. She thought it dreadful that the men had to live under His constant reproach.

DRJ: How do you get on with the Bolthole missionary zeal?

Mary was glad that I asked. Mrs Crispin (the headmistress) and Ivan are like that (she indicated by crooked fingers a degree of cozy intimacy). *They are both very religious. I find it hard not to scream in agony, but I don't because they'd only think I was Antichrist or something, and Ivan is marvelous. There's this missionary friend of Mrs. Crispin, a Miss Crabtree. They're always trying to drag her in, whether it fits into the scheme or not.*

This is interesting, and roughly corresponds with my own position. The continued spectacle of homo sapiens doing good to his fellow creature may be reassuring, but it lacks intellectual bite. What causes social problems in the first place?

(Enter Ivan Richards.) Ivan's response is surprisingly similar. He confesses an almost identical disquiet. Ivan: *I'm Church of England, you see. Now make no mistake about it, they're doing a wonderful job and one not easily done by people of other persuasions* (at this point, scribbling openly, I actually asked him to slow down, which he did obligingly and without question). *My own approach is liberal.*

He then moves on to his own diagnosis. The Army is "culturally deprived." It attracts "narrow people" who are "trapped in an attitude of mind." It all results in a "denial of legitimate pleasure." Why not (he wonders) art or music or decoration? Is the drabness really necessary?

We discussed total institutions and I tell them about Jim. Could the girls understand this kind of problem? They think that they could. DRJ will join the teaching team in the near future.

Some tentative conclusions:

Well, obviously an educative experience, but what came out of it?

1. A teaching opportunity. The depression felt by the girls needs to be pinned honestly and courageously to what they actually saw and not what they were expected to see.

2. Art work already organized with Betty Cranfield to give a painting to every man as a gesture on behalf for light and colour.

3. A very serious and extended appraisal by DRJ and the teachers that went on long after 4 P.M. What are the educational purposes of this kind of exercise? How can the different insights be organized and assessed? Is Mary a cynic? Is Ivan being defensive about his own religious image in the school? (He denied this one.) Is DJ a squalid nuisance, badgering the faithful? How can kids understand and test their own reactions? Why did different elements in the situation point so dramatically in different directions?

A pretty large ragbag of puzzles, and in the end, they were left for another day. Oh, I forgot to tell you. *The men are not allowed to smoke, except in the Gents.*

One could say that the Salvation Army did have a resonance here. David Jenkins struggled to find a balance between the care given to the needy and their subjugation to religious conformity. And raised in us the more general question: Is there always some such price to pay for kindness? Perhaps it's too much a prejudice to see the men housed and fed and working at the Ethel Street Hostel as needy. Did we force an unwarranted definition of humanism on the scene? Didn't they peel the potatoes for "theirselves?" It was a situation seen by an outsider, one who entertained the possibility that he was a nuisance and badgerer. Surely there was more to the situation than the Bolthole girls and David Jenkins were able to see. It is hard to say how much of our effort should be devoted to understanding the circumstances.

## REFERENCES

Brown T., B. (2019). *Holy envy: Finding God in the faith of others.* Harper-One.
Denny, T. (2016). *Being with the dying.* Mayhaven Publishing.
eukaryote. (2018). *The funnel of human experience.* LessWrong. https://www.lesswrong.com/posts/SwBEJapZNzWFifLN6/the-funnel-of-human-experience
Golden Rule. (n.d.). In *Wikipedia.* https://en.wikipedia.org/wiki/Golden_Rule
Harris, S., & Harris, A. (2013). *Lying.* Four Elephants Press.
Jenkins, D. R. (1969). "Saved by the Army." Internal report from the Keele Integrated Studies Project. In D. Hamilton, D. Jenkins, C. King, B. MacDonald, & M. Parlett (Eds.), *Beyond the numbers game.* MacMillan.
Stenhouse, L. (1973). The Humanities Curriculum Project. In H. R. Butcher & H. B. Pont (Eds.), *Race and education across cultures* (pp. 305–321). Heineman Educational Books.
Taylor Brown, B. (2019). *Holy envy: Finding God in the faith of others.* HarperCollins.

## NOTE

1. *The Bible,* English Standard Version, Romans 11:33.

# CHAPTER 5

# FREEDOM AND GOVERNING

> He let the phone slip from his hand and lay crying for a while, silently, shaking the cheap bed. He didn't know what to do, how to live. Each new thing he encountered in life impelled him in a direction that fully convinced him of its rightness, but then the next new thing loomed up and impelled him in the opposite direction, which also felt right. There was no controlling narrative: he seemed to himself a purely reactive pinball in a game whose only object was to stay alive for staying alive's sake.
>
> —Jonathan Franzen In *Freedom* (2010, p. 318)

A care paradigm probably would put care at the center of our lives and of our society. It could become the plot of our lives. It could give us a better sense of coherence, direction, of being governed by something that matters. A sense of belonging. A "Wirkungszuzammenhang," the German philosopher Hans-Georg Gadamer might call it.

A care paradigm is responsive to positions of precarity, fragility, and resilience. Governments, especially those in Western countries, recently under the banner of austerity, have been encouraging people to take care of, to care for, and to care about, one another, instead of relying on care provided by the government. The call for a society with a shared care ethic remains, for the most part, an "individualization" rally. People are still expected to manage their lives independently, and act as if their lives were an open project (Giddens, 1991). But Richard Morehouse and coauthors (2019) spoke with young adults, hearing:

I'm 22 and it feels like I'm still in my early 20s, or even late teens. It's like: When are you going to get a boyfriend? When are you going to have kids? When are you going to get married? When are you going to finish school? Have you finished school? What's your major? Where are you going to school? Where will you go to graduate school? Are you going for a doctorate? When are you going to get an adult job? Why is that not an adult job? Why are you going to work more hours? Oh, my God. Leave me alone. (p. 13)

The freedom (or necessity) to be an "entrepreneurial self" (Bröckling, 2015) puts pressure on people, especially on the younger generations. In *Sources of the Self*, Charles Taylor (1989) traced understanding of the self throughout history. He and others argue that our late-modern era has a focus on *self-realization*. Many of us are pressured to decide between competing choices to realize and govern our "self" (Beck & Beck-Gernheim, 2002).

## THE PRICE OF CHOICE

Anthony Giddens (1991) spoke of people living a "choice biography," a promise of freedom. But what happens when our efforts do not lead to good outcomes? Or when the unexpected, such as illness or loss of endeared holdings interrupt the plans? How do we care for ourselves? We may lose our sense of well-being, we may lose the security of being at ease in the world. If that happens, we enter a phase of disease, discomfort, of strangeness and unfamiliarity. Instead of being able to "flourish," or (more realistically) to live our lives as well as possible, Morehouse et al. (2019) argued that we are "floundering," struggling with anxiety and depression. That comfortable self-perception slips away.

At times all of us walk the brink. People's lives are precarious, even those more privileged. *Precarity* is not so much about being oppressed, but about feeling powerless against insecurity. Frans Vosman and Alistair Niemeijer (2017) wrote about precarity as: "the more subtle working of power [that] spreads insecurity that can engulf the lives of many, the seemingly dominant people as well" (p. 10). We *all* need protection and care, often different than those currently on offer. Sometimes we need care that controls and protects, other times a care that holds us, like an embrace. The latter is a form of care that is *relational:* determined not only by our own possibilities and capabilities, but also by the communities of which we are part. Morehouse et al. (2019) said:

We not only actively steer our lives as free agents, but we also "undergo" events and situations, evoked by larger patterns of traditions, regulations, evaluations and institutions. How we live our lives, how we determine next steps, does not happen against traditional, historically grown standards anymore, nor against clear ideas on what is "good and bad." (p. 13)

According to sociologists, this is the late-modern condition of society as a whole: the disappearance of certainty and tradition.

This uprooted social condition impacts how society is governed. In the United States, many collaborations are "bottom-up." Still we see a wide distinction between society and the bureaucracies. Hierarchical modes of governance remain dominant in many places. In Western Europe—before refugee flight and covid-19—many were the trends of less governmental control, sometimes moves to nonhierarchical modes of governing. This was stirred by failed reforms of policies, such as social and health care policies.

In Western Europe, especially the Northern countries, the gaps between citizens and the state were lessening, trending toward collaborative policy-making and social innovation. Governments, local and national, aimed to become "participatory" and self-regulated to develop policies and regulations supported by large numbers of citizens. Instead of making policies on the drawing table, policies were to be developed in close collaboration with stakeholders, implemented, tested and adjusted simultaneously. Incorporating citizen perspectives in how society and states are governed is in line with ideals such as solidarity, equity and trust: the three pillars of a *caring democracy* that Joan Tronto (2013) writes about in her book with the same title. We will get back to that after the following case.

Nothing is free of governance. Freedom fighters are governed. Honeymooners are governed. Governments are governed. Of course the range and benevolence of governance varies, from place to place and from time to time, and with more regard to some people and less to others. Some governance is the instrument of caring, and some is the obstacle to it. It can be both. Rare is the moment when one greatly dominates the other, freedom and governing, but we regularly feel the imbalance.

The agencies of governance are created to take care of matters. And in our personal lives we takes steps to control and protect our well-being, our own and that of others near and far. We pay too little attention to the side effects of governance, just as we do with the side effects of freedom. The freedom to bear arms, to drive while sleepy, to vote for pathologically deficient leaders, to write books about our cravings, these are freedoms that have a price. We would extend a care paradigm, only to find our cares are confrontational, a threat to others, a drag upon the futures of our children. Better planning might reduce some or all of the problem. There is no choice but to try, and then to try quickly to mitigate the blunders. It is another name for governing.

Tomas doesn't swear as much as he used to. But sometimes he embarrasses Marie. They agree that certain words should not be heard. They had been watching serials on Netflix, and heard too many of them. So they don't watch serials as much. Having just watched *L'Bureau*, we think it a high price to pay.

This next case tells of a U.S. Veteran Benefits Regional Office providing health and finanancial arrangements to veterans, clearly striving to improve their care.[1] The VA national leadership had been pressed by Congress to improve letters sent to veterans. Workshops were mandated for regional workers about Reader Focused Writing (RFW). Previously, legalities, bureaucratic requirements and indicators of production had had priority. The RFW training was thought well done by many staff members, but changes in letter-writing did not occur, not at the expense of caseload productivity.

## Indianapolis Regional Office

Robert Stake

Upstairs on the third floor of the Federal Building, I inquired about services to Indiana veterans. The workers there were aware that from time to time the federal Veterans Benefit Administration (VBA) was accused of writing incomprehensible letters. They knew from experience that over the years, many letters had been bad, filled with legal jargon and bureaucratic syntax. Furthermore, they knew that they were part of a political context. But when they discussed their work, they spoke consistently without reference to the media, Congressional oversight, or what the public thought of them. Theirs was a world of veterans, many of whom they had talked to on the phone, a world that included loan agencies, hospitals, and colleges. They referred often to the Central Office in Washington, but in organizational terms, not political.

**The Station.** The VBA Regional Office in Indianapolis provided services for disability compensation, pensions, vocational rehabilitation, and backing for home loans. Educational· and insurance benefits were handled at St. Louis and Cleveland, respectively. As the division names imply, these services are quite different, and specialized within, so that the responsibilities of different workers ranged greatly from room to room across the station. Staff size was about 145, down from a high of 200 three years earlier. Loan Guaranty currently had 30 positions; Vocational Rehabilitation and Counseling, 11. What had been the largest group had become larger, with 81 positions, as Compensation and Pension (C&P) merged with Veterans Services. C&P was where adjudicators and rating specialists acted upon claims for support due to physical disability resulting from military service. The reorganization brought with it the expectation that more personal communication practices, via telephone and face-to-face counseling, would reduce the heavy load of adjudication letterwriting (although paper trails would not disappear). The local work in Loan Guaranty was changing as Indianapolis became the national center for a portfolio loan program. Down-sizing (called "rightsizing" by some) meant not only a diminution of time available to handle a claim but an increase in claims handled at a national rather than regional center.

The director of the Regional Office was Dennis Wyant, heading the office since mid-1994 after many years in the Central Office where he had been national director of Vocational Rehabilitation and Counseling. Wyant held a doctorate in Education and was a certified rehabilitation counselor. Despite being legally blind, Wyant kept an eye personally on what was happening around the station. He was a "people person," a "problem-solver," neither confrontive nor authoritarian. He heard well what his chiefs and assistants had to say about running the programs. He expressed strong support of Reader Focused Writing as a step in the improvement of services to veterans.

Claims for benefits are made by veterans filling out forms. Most veterans have made contact with one of the service organizations, the American Legion and Veterans of Foreign Wars, for example, and many first encounter VBA with a form already filled in. Some requests are taken by telephone or over the counter, but quickly forms become the currency. Some forms are supplemented with records from doctors or campus admissions offices or county offices and such. The evidence is reviewed and a reply prepared. For a disability compensation claim, an adjudicator will recognize which on the menu of computer letters should be called up, and by using Microsoft Word and PCGL (Personal Computer Generated Letters) and by filling in blanks, modifying language, and attaching forms and pamphlets, compose a reply to the claimant.

A quality assurance review annually examines a sample of cases from the compensation and pension files, 106 were selected for 1996, of which 90 were reviewed by a federal team. Attention is given to the appropriateness of findings and not to the appropriateness of the communication. At Indianapolis, for a while, different divisions were conducting their own quality assurance operations but reports are no longer required and the practice waned.

**RFW Training.** On September 24, 1996, Wyant wrote to his division chiefs informing them of the RFW schedule as follows:

> We are nearing our scheduled time for Indianapolis to receive RFW training. Each RFW Tools Course consists of seven sessions; approximately

three hours each of core instruction and a 2–3 hour follow-up approximately 6-8 weeks following the class. The three hours per day includes two hours of broadcast instruction plus one hour of class. exercises and practice Since we have eight keypads, we can train eight during the morning and eight during the afternoon.

Such lengthy all-staff training had not happened previously at the station. Opposition to the plan among the chiefs and among the workers was considerable, voiced as putting too much strain on the workload, but also with skepticism that this professional development workshop, "as always before," one trainee said, would be anything more than consciousness-raising. It also was recognized that, for most of the participants, letter-writing to veterans was not a large part of their job description. But opposition melted with realization of the generality of the communication principles and the appeal of the composition techniques, warmed also by opportunity to work on interesting tasks with staffers from other divisions and by the high quality of the broadcasts. In retrospect, essentially all participants considered the training relevant, practice-changing, and personally upgrading.

For two hours a day in a· corner of the station's large conference room, the eight participants for each session watched—via satellite screen—Melodee Mercer, a loan guarantee specialist in Philadelphia and member of the VBA communications task force coaching the RFW and interacting on touch pads. "On page 48 of your manual, in the letter from Timothy Morrell, what implied questions can you identify? Your light is on, Frank at Detroit, what questions are implied in his letter?" The individual touch pad connections failed often, but ordinary phones then were substituted. The third hour was used for group activities. The exercises were well developed, thought-provoking, especially in that they gave the specialists opportunity to see how coworkers in other divisions resolved content problems. No further broadcasts were scheduled and even the six-week-later sessions disappeared.

**Obstacles to Implementation.** One of the primary findings from our fieldwork is that there was not a close match between the training and the actual work at Regional Offices. It has already been mentioned that the work is diverse and specialized, yet the training was the same for all participants.

Regional Office staff members who participate in VBA training in October, 1996, were unanimous in considering quality of letter-writing to veterans an important issue and that writers should strive to orient more to the veteran's needs. All of the 29 but two said that the VBA approach made sense to them and all but three said that VBA was *not* making too much of a fuss about improving letter writing.

In the interviews as well as in the surveys, it was apparent that the staffers supported a continuing effort to improve letter-writing. An interviewee said,

> It has been a long time since we have taken a hard look at letter writing and communication skills in general. The letters we used to use were confusing, legalistic. The Agency as a whole needed to provide the legal angle, and that still is the dominant attitude across the Agency. We were not able to advocate for the veteran, to gather information to advance his claim. RFW was the first time the Agency clearly provided a pro-veteran view. It was long overdue.

In interviews with six of these respondents, it was also apparent that they felt that the quality of letter writing had improved considerably in the last several years. When asked why, two or three said, "The main reason is that the standard computer letters that we draw from are much better than they were." Twenty-four indicated they had applied RFW ideas to their own work, four of those said "often."

We asked these 29 trainees what portion of their work time they presently spent writing letters to veterans. Nine of them indicated they did not do that at all and the median for the group was doing it only 5% of the time. Only three of them indicated that they spent half their time or more writing letters to veterans.

In two separate ways, we asked them the average amount of time in the last year spent on developing RFW skills. The median was 1–2 hours per month. Almost half of them had participated in earlier VBA efforts to improve letter writing. About a third of them had once had a formal writing improvement course. When asked about the need for in-service training of all kinds, the median of the group responses was that 4 hours a month should be set aside.

As to the training activity, 26 of the 29 checked that it was well organized. The same number said they learned much about better letterwriting. Just over half said the videos and materials were of high quality, five said low. About half of them said that the quality of the contribution of the on-site instructor was low.

As to implementation, 20 indicated that it was impractical to implement RFW in the ways illustrated in the course, apparently meaning that there were just very few occasions for start-from-scratch letter writing, and too little time to do it. When asked if the organization of the Regional Office had changed in any way to support RFW, 17 said "no" and another 11 said they did not know. In follow-up, they assured us that the officers had clearly indicated their support for RFW letter writing but, as they saw it, the organization had not changed to make it happen, and most did not see ways that it should change.

When asked if simpler letters trying to deal with a complex situation sometimes steer the veteran wrong, chiefs and workers alike said they could not identify cases of that happening. One added, "The complex information is in the attachments and we always tell them how to ask for more information."

One thing apparent in discussions at Indianapolis was a perceived mismatch between the training as designed and work methods and workload of the staff. The training apparently did not sufficiently acknowledge the diversity of communication responsibilities within VBA or sufficiently point to the generality of the RFW approach for communication in general. Two suggestions arising again and again were that in their own communications by letter, the Central Office should exemplify RFW and that the computer letters and the PCGL programs should be further upgraded along RFW lines.

**The Image of Service.** Even under careful probing, the staff of the Indianapolis Regional Office revealed a strong work ethic and a sincerity in being of service to Veterans. But they also were careful to maintain a good public image. They were highly aware of the low regard many citizens have for federal employees, and they themselves decried bureaucracy and political motive, for, in their own eyes, they were "Hoosiers," not bureaucrats.

Still they could not overlook the fact that in Oklahoma City, a federal services building of vintage and set-aside like theirs, had been blown apart. When I asked why the empty slot on the directory where earlier the Director's Office had been identified (Room 397) and when I asked why a punch-code lock on the door to the director's suite, I was told they were changed when an angry veteran had threatened Rowland Christian, the Assistant Director. In an age when citizens daily watch television actors acting out their rage, these public servants know that violence can quickly come to them.

But they also know all but a few of the thousands they serve are reasonable men and women seeking only their entitlements. They are aware that the laws awarding those benefits are complex but have a confidence that their legal and technical people have appropriately categorized the conditions that establish and differentiate eligibilities. They take pride in their efforts to communicate and feel that changes in rules and word processing in the last few years have made almost all of their letters comprehensible. They would like better form letters and even more training and work time to purge their letters of typographical errors, inconsistencies and obfuscations.

## MEASURING CARE

The RFW training, seen as high quality training, clashed with production quotas. It failed, although recognized as needed pro-veteran strategy, a better care advocacy for the veteran. Most of the Indianapolis staff undoubtably cared to be of service to the veterans, but they were also committed to caring for their jobs and the fiscal integrity of the federal agency. How is it that means-goals (bureaucracy, procedures) can become more important than end-goals (serving, advocacy)? The same choice occurs throughout society.

We live in a never-ending search for quality. Every minute's thought is a sensitivity to amounts of wellness, to the effects of youth and antiquity, to function and dysfunction, to goodness and badness, whatever merit. Edward Thorndike (1918), one of the fathers of modern psychology, asserted this pair of theses: "Thesis 6. Whatever exists at all, exists in some amount. Thesis 7. Anything that exists in amount can be measured." Measured badly sometimes, but in human belief and practice—measured, quantified, held dear.

Measurement governs much of our lives. Sometimes by choice, other times by rule or obligation. There are many apps on our smart phones that support the self-tracking of our bodies. Serious ones, such as measuring blood pressure or heart rate, and more playful ones such as for joggers counting the number of steps, and for parents of young viewers, their screen-time. In a study by Kappler et al. (2016), a young man confessed:

> Really, I've got a scale which analyses body fat and weight. Every day I use the scale. I do not use it Mondays, it is too shocking, because you have just passed the weekend (laughing), and that causes such a peak, which is not realistic; but on Tuesday I exercise. I had a reasonable Monday, and on Wednesday morning I can reuse my scale without further concerns. Everything is normal again (laughing). (p. 77)

He also explains how he plays with measurements and conventions, comparing his body mass index and body fat. Another person, Kate, is much more interested in "beautiful" results. If she gets a number that she doesn't like, she "walks around the block, in order to obtain a "beautiful" round or curious figure. She also wanted to get nice tracks on the maps: "nicely shaped forms" and to never walk the same path twice, because that generates "silly pictures." This suggests again that well beyond clocks and speedometers, people's lives are governed by measurement tools. Freely chosen, much of the time, but making us less free than we realize. It may even steal from our bodily wisdom and sensitivity:

> B: And then you think, I should have a defect. And you look for symptoms.... Well, and I simply turned off my own thinking.
>
> I: Yeah.

B:   Yes, and my knowledge, what I already had … and I
completely trusted that what was presented there, reflected
what was really wrong with me. And that was not true.

A carpenter's memory is fixed: "Measure twice and cut once." We all are
carpenters of one sort or another. We make things. We fix things. We care
for things. But we haven't cared enough about fixing the world so that
its peoples, its creatures, its lands and its oceans, live good lives. Seeking
the solidarity. Seeking the resonance. We have a need to nourish a more
universal care paradigm.

In our world, many are the instances of negligence and malpractice. But
the people of the world provide a vast radiance of love, protection, sacrifice
and uplifting. Yet most of the radiance extends to family and affinity, falling
short of the care needed broadly and further out. Bad caretaking, person to person, is the smaller problem, important but acknowledged. The
super-perplexing problem is the lack of restraint thrust forth to counter
the greater social intrusions, from poverty to discrimination to disinterest
in the environment and to abuse and to violence.

Researchers, social advocates, masters of language and communication,
as opposed to those on the front line, they (we) have special obligations
to nourish a care paradigm. We write, we critique, we explore the media,
and we teach. And we ignore much that needs highlighting. And there is
no greater need for nourishment than in the instruction we give and the
evaluation we do of societal needs, services, and programs. No inventions,
no new networks, no prerequisites are needed. We are asking ourselves to
think, upon every minute's encounter with values: "Here, right now: Is care
adequately present?"

Are we ready? A line in one of the old Western movies went, "A glass on
the table in case a bottle swims by?" What constitutes us being ready?

Time given to care, money spent on care, hugs given back to care, can
be counted. But full care, full quality of care, can neither be counted nor
measured directly. Psychometrics can provide indirect measures, attempts
at correlates of care, but these measures have lacked and will continue to
lack validity. Still, imperfectly, yet persuasively, we do *experience* volume and
worth of care. With observation and questioning, we can get good estimates
of care offerings. Were they meticulously aggregated, we could have local
and national indicators of care. Would they be worth it? Would they be used
to improve policies? We doubt it. Better to spend the money on care itself.

But to return to the second to last paragraph. We do not need to have
a good psychometric or econometric indicator of care in order to ask the
question, "In this activity, the one we are looking at right now, is care
adequately present?" Just raising the question matters. We upgrade the

expectation that it is something that needs more attention. We work for a strengthened care paradigm. We should have it on the tip of our tongues: "Is the idea of caring prominent in this place?" Thinking about that starts in our earliest years.

## PLAYING AND REALITY

When even in our early years, we get glimpses of what care is and is not. Even before we were born, we were dependent upon our mothers. Once stepping out unhanded, our parents set rules, restrictions, and left us free to play. Being protected too much may stir a fear of domination, being left too free may make us careless too.

Donald Winnicott (1964) said that to have a "healthy" society, we need to accept our earliest dependencies. We need to acknowledge the devotion of mother and father to their children. When this devotion is off balance, too much or too little, once grown up, people may avoid being dominated, and they may be drawn towards another chosen authority. By ignoring or denying the dependency of the child upon its parents, Winnicott thought that a fear is instilled in the child that has repercussions for society as a whole: the fear of being dependent. But dependence is biological, emotional, and as human as it can be. We are dependent upon others, we are dependent upon that that surrounds us: others, objects, abstract numbers, agreements.

Being governed by our dependencies, is part of everyday reality. It lays the seeds for caring human beings. Dependency is not bad, not trivial. It is not something that needs to be resolved, but we need to learn how to relate to those dependencies in a healthy way. When society delays fully acknowledging dependency, complete health is interfered with. It may result in people who want to control, dominate, govern others. Worse, Winnicott argued, this fear may even take the form of a fear of care itself, as the mother is often associated with care, and at other times will take on less easily recognizable forms, always including the fear itself. Winnicott may be correct. This fear may start in the microspheres of childhood. He may also be mistaken. As when we grow up, we are surrounded by others who educate us, guide us toward other ways of relating, toward being governed, toward being free.

## REFERENCES

Franzen, J. (2010). *Freedom.* Farrar, Straus and Giroux.
Beck, U., & Beck-Gernheim, E. (2002). *Individualization: Institutionalized individualism and its social and political consequences.* SAGE.

Bröckling, U. (2015). *The entrepreneurial self: Fabricating a new type of subject.* SAGE.

Giddens, A. (1991). *Modernity and self-identity: Self and society in the late modern age.* Stanford University Press.

Kappler, E. K., Krzeminska, A., & Noji, E. (2018). Resonating self-tracking practices? Empirical insights into theoretical reflections on a "sociology of resonance. In B. Ajana (Ed.), *Metric culture: Ontologies of self-tracking practices* (pp. 77–99). Emerald.

Morehouse, R., Visse, M., Singer-Towns, B., & Vitek, J. (2019). Juggling the many voices inside: What it means to be an emerging adult. *International Journal of Psychological Research and Reviews, 2*(1), 1–18.

Stake, R. & Davis, R. (1999). Summary of evaluation of reader focused writing for the Veterans Benefits Administration. *American Journal of Evaluation.*

Stake, R., & Visse, M. (forthcoming). *Case sudy. International Encyclopedia of Education.* Elsevier.

Taylor, C. (1989). *Sources of the self: The making of the modern identity.* Cambridge UniversityPress.

Tronto, J. S. (2013). *Caring democracy: Markets, equality and justice.* NYU Press.

Thorndike, E. L. (1918). The nature, purposes, and general methods of measurements of educational products. In G. M. Whipple (Ed.), *The seventeenth yearbook of the National Society for Study of Education* (Part II. p. 16). Public School Publishing Company.

Vosman, F., & Niemeijer, A. (2017). *Rethinking critical reflection on care: late modern uncertainty and the implications for care ethics.* Medicine, Health Care and Philosophy. https://doi.org/10.1007/s11019-017-9766-1

Winnicott, D. (1964). *The child, the family and the outside world.* Pelican Books.

## NOTE

1. The CIRCE report to the U.S. Veterans Benefits Administration (1993) included this Indianapolis Regions Office case study (Stake, Davis, & Guynn, 1977). It was included in a professional paper by Robert Stake and Rita Davis (1999) and will be included in the 2022 edition of Elsevier's International Encyclopedia of Education.

# CHAPTER 6

# EMPATHY AND RECIPROCITY

In his book, *The Unknown Potential of the Everyday*, the Dutch chaplain and care ethics advisor Michael Kolen examines moral meanings in everyday interactions between young people with a mild intellectual disability (MID) and care professionals (Kolen, 2017). His research took place at the Prisma Foundation in The Netherlands, an organization for people with MID. The origins of that foundation date back to the 1904 Roman-Catholic order of friars. The friars wondered how people with an intellectual disability might live their lives together with other citizens. More than a century later, this question remains significant. There is a growing number of people with mild intellectual disability who cannot keep up the accelerating pace of our society (Rosa, 2010). It is not just this group experiencing increased precariousness. Research shows that depression is one of the most common disorders in the United States. Perhaps we, as a society, put demands on people too high. For many, just getting through the day matters most.

Showing and practicing empathy for those who are more precarious than we are is important. Empathy is being concerned about how another person is feeling. It extends to realizing how others are poorly fitting into their situations. With empathy we show compassion, as best we can, avoiding being paternalistic and overbearing. Empathy is a disposition, a character trait, a virtue that can be either cultivated and grown, or neglected and disregarded.

---

*a Paradigm of Care*, pp. 67–77

## DISPLACEMENT

In care ethic circles, empathy and compassion are forms of *displacement*. Usually we think of displacement as having to move to a different place, not wanting to, and feeling a loss of security, such as the monstrous displacement of U. S. Indian tribes (listen to Chief Joseph in Chapter 9). In care ethics, displacement is a positive term meaning movement toward recognition of the condition of another being. It comes with willingness to be repositioned toward fuller reception of the other's experience. But it is a movement without diminishing the experiencing of one's self. Were we to fuse ours with the other's experience—no longer having separate self-experience—it would not be empathy, but identification or entrainment (Ganczarek et al., 2018).

> It wasn't so long ago that Marie went to a Women's March. She told Tomas, "It was like something I never experienced before." Tomas said, "I wish I could have been there too." She said, "I wish that too, but I don't really think you could have had my experience."

Empathy does not come without problems. In a complex situation it can be simplistic, unidimensional, blunt. Some argue that empathy is an illusion because we are too little capable of seeing *beyond* the other's suffering and pain. They argue that we cannot simply turn off our interpretations and projections. Assumptions about others sooner or later will be wrong. But misconceptions or not, they do not necessarily reduce the powerful effect that empathy can evoke.

As we said in Chapter 4, there is a problem with the golden rule. The same problem exists with empathy. Empathy too can be presumptuous and potentially harmful, supposing that how *you* want to be treated is how others should be treated. Clearly some of the time, that presumption is a generous point of view. But it may be offering, even imposing, a set of values that do not fit the others.

It could be something like mandating a health care system for people who need better care but not recognizing what they would be forced to give up some of their present arrangement. The plan would provide some combination of gain and loss, not just gain or loss alone. Some of the onus diminishes as the situation is negotiable, that people can let you know how they would like to be treated. That recognition is what displacement means here.

## CHOICE

Choice is an essential social condition. Even if many choices are not available, some sense of ability to make choices, some critical choices, is important to our personal well-being. There always are limits. If healthy people are not obligated to participate in the health plan, then the costs go up, and benefits are limited. What should we do when people do not act in the best interests of the community, or even in their own best interests?

Individualized choices can be wonderful, especially for children. But a school system that offers an individualized curriculum for each child, often overlapping, but each decided largely on the uniqueness of the child, finds it much more expensive than the one *lehrplan* we have. The individualized plan is an overly demanding way to teach for many teachers. On the other hand, standardization of the curriculum is not defensible on what is best for society, partly because so little of it is challenging and providing lasting preparation. But what else could be offered with the resources available.[1] Considerably more individualization could occur if needs and appetites were more carefully assessed and cared about.

Needs and appetites are difficult to assess, not just those of children with disabilities but of all the children, and teachers, families, communities, and nations. Doing unto others as they would like done to themselves, is not a perfect target. Worse, it is beyond our assessment skills. Making things a little better, though, would be much better. Some addition of long-term tracking, staying in touch, keeping notes, should occur. Opportunity for correction, large and small choices, should be a feature of our improved golden rule and our optimized empathy.

A great part of the problem is the belief that the well-being of people is common to all, that people's needs and yearnings are universal. A quick look at lifestyles tells us sometimes that is largely not so. Unfortunately, in taking care of people, we have a strong motto: *one size fits all.* As it stands, getting it as cheap as possible and as profitable to the providers means stocking as few sizes as possible.

One view of empathy, and of humanism as well, is that people are seriously treated as needing to have more choices, more room to expand, more enjoyment of their uniquenesses, than they now have. Perhaps the standard should be that there is less standardization in the contexts of living. But if put to a vote, most of those below standard could be expected to vote for greater homogeneity. Still, there need not always be a choice between more choices and better accommodations

## FINDING PLACE

Michael Kolen pointed out that for people with mild intellectual challenge, interaction of everyday life can be a trial. They have hopes and dreams and wants and needs, but they keep finding themselves at the edge of things, of society, of their jobs, their social circle. Everyone wants to be better understood, cared for, and belonging somewhere. Kolen called this the process of *finding place* (Kolen, 2017). He writes that together in the kitchen, preparing a meal, peeling potatoes, can enhance one's sense of self and generate a sense of belonging. Being part of a community that cares, or an institution that cares, directly affects the everyday experience of living a life as well as possible. At the Prisma Foundation on Estate Assisië in the South of The Netherlands, artist studios for and exhibitions by people with disabilities are a common feature. Artistic expressions here and elsewhere serve to counterbalance the monoculture of verbal discourse and professional nomenclature of their lifeworld. Spaces for artistic experimentation at Prisma provide them with opportunity to access and share their lives with "others." Nonverbal modes of expression (under the guidance of creative therapists or not), can do justice to the different modes of knowing the world.

Not everyone is capable of finding the right words or joining the professional discourse. Not everyone is self-reliant or capable of being the citizen too often expected of us. We are vulnerable. Others who are able and willing to empathize with that sensitivity, understand that at times the world is overwhelming. With understanding comes the power to create safer

**Figure 6.1**

*Finding Place in the Kitchen*

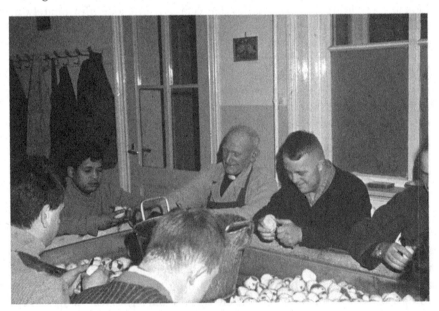

spaces for those who need them. At Prisma, this sensitivity has become the breeding ground for social innovation. There, new forms of togetherness, of being in community with different others and unaccustomed things, can unfold.

## RECIPROCITY

In addition to the formal conceptions of society in terms of the roles and positions we share, we need community.[2] We need to nurture the social ties that gathered people have with one another. In Kolen's (2017) case study, a professional care organization forged new coalitions with societal partners, such as artist collectives, private ventures and commercial parties, to invent new modes of care. He illustrated, beyond persons, how institutions and society can be better caregivers. Health care organizations broaden their scope by partnering with commercial parties. Sometimes it happens for economic reasons, sometimes even to survive financially, other times because of deeply held values and beliefs in a better society, a caring society.

These commercial initiatives may seem to be in contrast with the everydayness of personal living together. In his study, Kolen (2017) regularly mentioned how young people with mild intellectual disabilities are perceived to be "an annoyance" to others. They do not withhold from knocking on your door while you are in a meeting or when you have hung the "silence please" sign on your door. Nor do "these kids" act according to what we generally think is "appropriate" social conduct. In another study, the Dutch researcher Gustaaf Bos wrote about a challenging encounter with someone with severe intellectual disabilities. His name was Harry. Bos said: "After a while, I realized that I foremost felt deeply unable to respond adequately to Harry. Why did he approach me like this? What could he mean? What did he want from me? Moreover, how was I supposed to communicate with him in a reciprocal way?" (Bos & Abma, 2018).

Communicating with people who differ from ourselves can be a challenge. Instead of empathic, we may feel uneasy, even frustrated. When a care agency helps people, what is meant by reciprocity?

### A Religious Minority

Dannel McCollum (2020)

In 1943, Reverend Philip Schug was called to be minister of the Unitarian Church of Champaign-Urbana, Illinois. He circulated a newsletter to persons who somehow had identified themselves as having no religious

preference, identifying issues of concern, including upcoming state legislation officially permitting a somewhat common practice, the teaching of
sectarian religious education in public schools.

Vashti McCollum, a former law student and mother of three, answered
the invitation and followed Schug's suggestion to send letters to legislators
protesting such a bill. The replies from three local legislators told her not
to worry. Her oldest child, James, began the fifth grade the same year that
the Champaign School District's program in religious education, conducted by teachers hired by local churches, came to teach his grade and his
classroom.

Although it was a voluntary program, nonparticipants were to leave the
room during instruction. James, the only nonparticipant, had to leave the
classroom during the religious class. He was teased and shunned by class-
mates and over the long haul, made to feel singled out and uncomfortable.
Vashti, an atheist, angry about the discrimination, decided to file a lawsuit
against the school district. Schug offered his support and found additional
support for her in Chicago political and legal circles.

John Franklin, the school board attorney, advised Ms. McCollum that
if she proceeded with the case, she would become very unpopular in the
community. It was unfriendly advice. A local newspaper, the *Courier* ran a
long commentary by Schug about the lawsuit, detailing the Constitutional
separation of "church and state," agreement in the state constitution, and
a summary of problems in teaching religion in the public schools. Schrug's
opinion received no apparent support in town, and probably stirred hostil-
ity toward Vashti McCollum and her son.

The Illinois House passed the legislation with only two votes opposed.
Schug wrote a five-page paper to members of the Senate, emphasizing they
were dealing with a "very hot potato." He placed a copy of the paper on
each member's desk on the morning of the vote, and suddenly it became a
hot debate. When the vote came, opponents from Chicago and advocates
from Champaign were strong in the galleries. By close vote, the bill was
defeated. In the eyes of many of the community, it was a case of atheism
versus religion.

The lawsuit was taken up by the District Court. Asked if he believed in
God, Schug answered that God was seen differently by people, some of
whom he agreed with but until science could settle it, he would not want to
say. James' testimony as to his isolation was more persuasive to the specta-
tors. But the three judges turned down the petition. The Illinois Supreme
Court affirmed the ruling of the District Court. The United States Supreme
Court reversed the decision, ruling 8–1, that the Champaign religious education program was in violation of the U.S. Constitution.

The high majority of the local community had seen no reason to oppose
the school board's decision to include religious education in the curriculum. It is reasonable to conclude that they saw it as caring for the children,
providing them with knowledge and guidance for living. The supporters
of Vashti McCollum saw their position as one of caring for the children,

endorsing their freedom of worship and freedom from derision. It is not unusual for conflict to occur among caring people.

Our empathy does not arise from nowhere: it is a motivational displacement of oneself partially into another, which is aimed at understanding how it feels to be wrapped into what the other is experiencing. We take another's perspective, but—as mentioned previously—we still hold onto our own perspective. In some situations, we need to make more than a little effort to connect with the experiential world of the other. In other situations, it happens naturally.

Empathy is an outreach of care, but, still, it can cause lapses in ethical judgment. Lots of people empathize with outlaws such as Robin Hood and Butch Cassidy. We remember the Stockholm Syndrome. Studies about terrorists whose victims are "brainwashed," relate with empathy too. In many cases, a problematic empathy emerges less from shared aggression toward outsiders but from loyalty to insiders.

Empathy is not only about us displacing ourselves. We need the other to be displaced too. It is a reciprocal process. The other person needs to grant us access to his or her lifeworld. But only a partial access can be expected. How do we displace ourselves when the other person grants too little access? We do not always speak the language of the other, the immigrant, the alcoholic, the workmate calling for help, a call we fail to comprehend. Our empathy may impose a strange, threatening world on him or her. The impending decisions intended to be caring, may not appear so. Our imagination or presumptions work overtime. The call of the other, perhaps a call for care from suffering or some mysterious dark, may be interpreted wrongly, and draw a wrong response.

## SUFFERING

Empathy is well meant, but too much empathy, woven into caretaking, can ignore the labor of suffering. We show empathy and we position ourselves to alleviate someone's suffering. The joking, the cuddling, the opened window, may ignore the suffering. In many cases what was said to be helpful, is not. In some cases, being in pain—physical, emotional, spiritual—can be a productive endeavor that moves toward relief. An unanticipated, previously unknown relief. Too much empathy, too much caretaking, may take away the struggle with suffering. In general, we strive to reduce suffering. We perceive it as an undesired state needing to be resolved as quickly as possible. Suffering is a burden, widely treated as a dysfunction needing to be fixed. Are we wrong?

The prevailing view of suffering is closely related to how we, as a society, view the body and its senses. They are seen as instrumentalities, tools. They do not have inherent meaning simply because they exist as part of our identity. In public life, only a little space is given to the sensory dimensions of life. Verbal and measurable expressions prevail over sensory ways of knowing and being in the world. Our *aesthetic being*, our sensory world, remains largely unseen. Suffering is felt, but it is part of the world unseen.

Usually, aesthetic experience is perceived as something for an elite: for people privileged to enjoy the beauties of life. But aesthetics as a sensory approach to the world is not only about beauty. On an earlier occasion, we wrote about how aesthetics goes beyond "sensing" as in seeing solely with the eyes. Empathy is one of the other seeings. For empathy, the senses are necessary, but beyond them is still an "unknown." The following poem illustrates how aesthetics is not only about our sensory experience, referring to touch, smell, seeing and hearing, but one that moves into an experience that we can only bring deep into mind.

### Male Nurse Washing a Nun

by Geoffrey Bowe (2003)

Today
he had washed a nun.
She didn't seem to mind because he was doing his job. Her body
looked pale and unused,
her nipples
like the pile of stones
found at the summit of mountains. He talked to her
about *The Sound of Music*
as he washed her thighs.
"I know all the songs," she said. He asked her to roll over
so that he could wash her back and bottom
as they discussed Mother Teresa. For ten minutes
the sponge licked at her body as a ray of light
entered like an angel
through the gap in her curtains, illuminating the bed and its contents.
The male nurse noticed
how the pattern on the curtains looked like stained glass,
her bedside table like an altar.
He found himself kneeling down, beside the bed,
before pulling himself together
and leaving.

Aesthetics goes all the way back to the Greek *aisthesis* (sense perception) and *aisthetikos* (sensitive, perceptive). It integrates affective, motor, and sensory capacities. Maurice Merleau-Ponty (1962) wrote that these lived understandings arrive through our bodily being in the world, and through the sensations forming our experiences. The nursing assistant feeding a patient, or the male nurse washing the nun: both take us into the realm of conscious or tacit sensory experience. *Reading* about these experiences might evoke a sensory experience too. Something may seem to have been there, but we could not fully grasp it. Empathy is an aesthetic experience (for more see Ganczarek et al., 2018).

Something similar occurs when we feel empathy with someone's suffering. Its meaning cannot fully be known nor translated by the witness, tied as it is to human existential meaning. Our somatic-sensory world may connect us in ways that we cannot verbalize but is meaningful beyond measure and our power of explanation. Suffering, here, may be seen as a pathway leading to connection and compassion, and empathy.

The example of the nurse washing the nun, and other examples in this book show that some people know what it is to suffer in solidarity. Suffering in solidarity is a togetherness, a kind of togetherness that only emerges when sharing the hurt and the pain of another. Here, suffering generates reciprocity, a mutuality of care and understanding. Simply "receiving" the story and the trust of someone who suffers is a reciprocal act. Witnessing the hurt or vulnerability of another protects us from indulging in self-pity and being engrossed in our own misery. Instead, we think about others and come up with what we may be able to do to alleviate their pain, disease, or discomfort. In this way, we also help ourselves.

Nowadays, people hesitate to openly share pain, although the covid-19 crisis seems to change that. People who do not openly share their suffering may feel ashamed, afraid, or believe that they are responsible for themselves, especially in a Western neoliberal climate. Many hearts are over-defensive, closed, afraid to fully feel the pain, or troubled to ask another one for what they really need. Some blame others for not sensing those needs, but how can others know? Can we? How to sense the distress of another? Some know how to probe; ask the right questions. They can practice patience for the response that rings true to emerge. Only then does suffering become togetherness: when that time is taken when the process can unfold.

In situations of injustice the suffering increases. Even when carried together, this suffering has "added pain," it cannot be taken away, resolved, its powerlessness can only be carried and welcomed, felt completely, and transform into something else. All suffering may grow into renewed openness, the capacity to care, to reach out to others who need us. People who know how to care, how to practice kindness and compassion, first knew suffering. Naomi Shihab Nye (1995) captured that in the poem that ends the introduction to this book.

## EMPATHY AND THE IMAGINATION

The experience of sharing in others' suffering is not one-sided. Recently, care ethicists have dubbed empathy as a cocreative practice (van Dijke et al., 2020). In their article on relational empathy, Jolanda van Dijke and her coauthors (2020) quoted a chaplain who told them about one of his clients guiding him *through* his experience of moving into a small studio apartment in a rehabilitation center: "Then my client says to me: 'Imagine.... Imagine this is happening to you.'" He points to the room where he sits.... He says: "This entire space is smaller than my study room at home." And then he points to the kitchen block and says: "That would be my kitchen. That shelf, that would be my cellar. My bathroom. Bedroom. Office." Turning to the interviewer the chaplain says: "I see something happening to you now that I tell you this.... What happens, I think, is that we can finally imagine what it is like" (p. 4).

Here, next to establishing a relationship with each other, the story evokes an imaginary space that the listener is invited to enter. We cannot empathize with another without accessing our imagination or that imaginary realm. This is basically what the field of Narrative Medicine is about: narration as a means to raise physician empathy. By close reading and by reflective writing, physicians and other health professionals are invited to step into the imaginary world of a protagonist. By training narrative competence, clinical imagination and clinical empathy, readers develop attentiveness, tuning into patients' experiences. They learn to listen deeply to what is buried in a story, not just the surface, the plot, the critical moments, but they are trained to "listen" to bodily gestures, silences, metaphors, genres, and allusions. Virginia Woolf (1932) once wrote: "Open your mind as widely as possible, then signs and hints of almost imperceptible fineness ... will bring you into the presence of a human being unlike any other" (p. 259). She also wrote: "To read a novel is a difficult and complex art. You must be capable not only of great fineness of perception, but of great boldness of imagination" (p. 259). One need not have experienced the suffering or fate of the other, to empathize with him or her, and to help. Learning how to read vicariously may foster this. Some call this the aesthetic approach, as we live through something of the same experiences as the protagonist. Some call this narrative medicine. More often we call it caring.

## REFERENCES

Bos, G., & Abma, T. (2018). Responding to otherness: the need for experimental-relational spaces. In M. Visse & T. Abma (Eds.), *Evaluation for a caring society* (pp. 159–185). Information Age Publishing.

Bowe, G. (2003). Male nurse washing a nun. In C. Davis & J. Schaefer (Eds.), *Intensive care: More poetry & prose by nurses.* University of Iowa Press.

Dijke, J. van Nistelrooij, I. van, Bos, P., & Duyndam, J. (2020). Towards a relational conceptualization of empathy. *Nursing Philosophy, 21,* 3. https://doi.org/10.1111/nup.12297

Ganczarek, J., Hünefeldt, T., & Olivetti Belardinelli, M. (2018). From "Einfühlung" to empathy: exploring the relationship between aesthetic and interpersonal experience. *Cognitive Process, 19,* 141–145.

Kolen, M. (2017). *The unknown potential of the everyday.* Proefschriftmaken.

Rosa, H. (2010). *Acceleration and alienation: Towards a critical theory of late-modern temporality.* NSU Press.

McCollum v. Board of Educ., 333 U.S. 203 (1948).

Merleau-Ponty, M. (1962). *Phenomenology of perception* (C. Smith, Trans.). The Humanities Press.

Shihab Nye, N. (1995). *Words under the words: Selected poems* (A Far Corner Book). The Eighth Mountain Press.

Woolf, V. (1932). *How should one read a book?* In A. McNeillie (Ed.), *The common reader* (p. 259). Hartcourt.

## NOTES

1. In 2020, the *New York Times* devoted several articles to individualized school learning. See: https://www.nytimes.com/topic/subject/education-and-schools
2. Here, we refer to the traditional distinction between the German Gemeinschaft and Gesellschaft (see https://en.wikipedia.org/wiki/Gemeinschaft_and_Gesellschaft)

# CHAPTER 7

---

# COMPETITION AND GRACE

---

Not all of us are super-competitive; some are. A lot of us have our favorite teams, especially if one of our own is on the team. We know that it can be a precious experience when the team is working together, of course, to beat the brains out of opponents. And to have a caring coach, and there is no requirement that he or she teaches sportsmanship all the time.

When a mom yells, "Knock'm back to the fifth grade!" or when a team-mate asks, "You ready to whack Big Shot down a notch?," we know we have not climbed the caring mountain. Yes, in winning we satisfy the lust for taking care of the team, momentarily.

The caring ethic does not have the mission of ending competition. There is zero chance that dressing up or pie baking or even documentary watching will ever be free of competition. But caring could move up the scale quite a bit without trying to take the lust out of gaming. Just taking a quarter the pain out of math class or pharmaceutical advertising would be a step in the right direction. But we need more than that.

Writer James Carse (1986) wrote that there are two kinds of games. One is played for the purpose of winning. It has an end and a beginning, a win-ner and loser. It has rankings and stars and rules. The other game is for the purpose of continuing the play. It is infinitely long and has no eligibility conditions: everyone can play. Anyone may join. The rules can change if it helps continue the play. This game needs care for more than winning and losing; it cares about playing the game. Marriage and car repair and police protection are such games.

---

*a Paradigm of Care*, pp. 79–91

But most recognized gaming is the first kind, a power play. And all can play. Even the poorest of us has the power to allocate privilege. With warm smiles and sincere attention, we help make other lives more livable. With carelessness and honor roles we make other lives less livable. Alas, our social policies only work to make life more livable for some, and less livable for others. How dare we discriminate so!

It is super-apparent in schools. Let us look carefully for a few moments at the classroom situation. Everyone knows that schools are not the benevolent, personally supportive, humanistic places they could be. And should be. Our views of talent, equity, and course grading in schools influence the perceptions, including self-perceptions, of children and all of us. We mold ourselves, grading, pushing ourselves up the ladder and others down. Standardized testing and teacher testing, in particular, needlessly hurtfully facilitate an academic caste system, often thought to be in the best long-run interests of the participants. Most teachers will say, "No, it is best care for the children, and the rest of us, to make us more competitive, to make winners.

## TALENT

In the 1930s, Nebraska, as other states, held State Fairs that had rodeos and animal judging and yes, baby contests. Ribbons and silver cups were given for the "healthiest." The announced purpose of the contest was to examine the health of drought-years children, mostly rural, many not being regularly seen by a doctor. What could be a better example of caring?

Just south of there, at the Kansas State Fair, another purpose of the competition was framed on the clinic wall, something like: "to discourage breeding in families of inferior talent." The international Eugenics Society was behind the posters. That was about the time Adolph Hitler was running for Chancellor of Germany.

In Paris, more than a century ago, the government first called for the measurement of talent, particularly intelligence, even more particularly, scholastic aptitude. Psychologist Alfred Binet, studying mental function, was commissioned by the French government to create a test to weed out children in school unable to learn at a "normal" pace.

The test did discriminate, almost to world satisfaction, with few people questioning. But an item of the Simon-Binet test is shown here, asking, for each pair, "Which of these two faces is the prettier?" (see Figure 7.1).

Seventy years later, John Flanagan, a University of Pittsburgh psychometrician, created Project Talent (Flanagan, 1960). Testing 400,000 U.S. kids annually, he sought talent among the nation's youth. But—as so many social science studies go—the interest in helping people gave way to interest in finding correlation of variables. The research mostly promoted additional research. Would this have been more humane had it

**Figure 7.1**

*Pictures for Binet-Simon Scale*

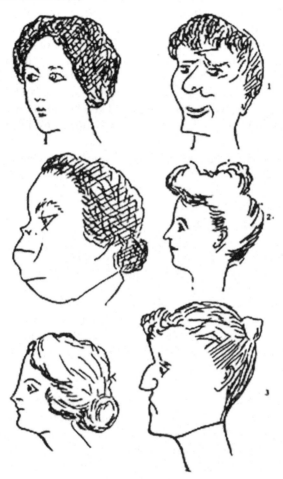

been commissioned in the humanities rather than the social sciences? It is difficult to see today's humanistic studies as more caring than the social sciences? Either one, for that matter.

## MORE ON EQUITY

The major approaches for studies of equity (Scriven, 1993) are said to be choices between formative and summative evaluation, but that needs be twisted only a quarter around to be between a search for quality of the process versus quality of the results. Similarly, advocacy of equity can be for bettering the process or product, and it can be less for action and more for comprehension, comprehension in general or in a particular context. An advocate can strive for taking action or only to strengthen a point of view. Equity needs a consideration of the situation, a commitment to fairness and an understanding of quality.

In Chapter 1 we wrote about equity, particularly about inequities of grading and testing in the schools. We claimed that repetitiously confronting a person with his or her low standing among other persons, even though considered necessary, was discriminatory, unfair, and an act of poor care. The legitimacy of such discrimination has been bolstered by the technology of mandated and standardized testing. We want to examine this inequity further here.

In 1960, Henry Chauncey was president of the Educational Testing Service (ETS) in Princeton, NJ. ETS had made some of the best standardized tests for measuring verbal and math scholastic aptitude, particularly for college admissions. But Chauncey was embarrassed by the narrowness of this definition of talent, and urged his researchers to broaden their views (Lemann, 2001). At one meeting (that one of us attended), they discussed a new personality inventory, the Myers-Briggs Type Indicator, authored by two women, Katherine Briggs and Isabel Myers. It was based on the Jungian idea that persons were highest on one of four psychological functions: sensation, intuition, feeling, or thinking. Measuring *these* functions might lead to better recognizing the complexity of talent and aspiration and the opportunity for individualized instruction. But the researchers at the meeting were adamant in their assessment that the validity of Myers-Briggs was low. Their question was not, "Would it help?" but "Is it precise enough?" (see Figure 7.2).

Twenty years later, a distinguished testing man, Lee Cronbach tried for a decade to find a "talent platform" on which more differentiated learning and behavior might be based (Cronbach & Snow, 1997). He called it, aptitude-treatment interaction. "Teach *each* to his or her individual talent." After several years, he gave up saying, "I'm sure it's there; we just couldn't find it."

Over the years, Joel Spring, an educational philosopher, wrote numerous books about national educational policy. One book was *The Sorting Machine* (1988) in which he claimed the primary aim of the schools was to identify and favor the children fitting-best the U.S. economic structure.

## SORTING

Societally, is sorting needed? Pedagogically, is tracking needed? Educationally, are tests needed? Standardized tests provide ranks of students. They

**Figure 7.2**

*A Chart With Descriptions of Each Myers-Briggs Personality Type and the Four Dichotomies Central to the Theory. Detail on the Web*

# What's Your Personality Type?

| ISTJ | ISFJ | INFJ | INTJ |
|---|---|---|---|
| Inspector | Protector | Counselor | Mastermind |
| Doing What Should Be Done | A High Sense of Duty | An Inspiration to Others | Everything Has Room for Improvement |
| **ISTP** | **ISFP** | **INFP** | **INTP** |
| Crafter | Composer | Healer | Architect |
| Ready to Try Anything Once | Sees Much But Shares Little | Performing Noble Service to Aid Society | A Love of Problem-solving |
| **ESTP** | **ESFP** | **ENFP** | **ENTP** |
| Promoter | Performer | Champion | Inventor |
| The Ultimate Realist | You Only Go Around Once in Life | Giving Life an Extra Squeeze | One Exciting Challenge After Another |
| **ESTJ** | **ESFJ** | **ENFJ** | **ENTJ** |
| Supervisor | Provider | Teacher | Fieldmarshal |
| Life's Administrators | Hosts and Hostesses of the World | Smooth-talking Persuader | Life's Natural Leaders |

do not tell what a student knows. They do not tell what a student can do. All they do is sort students, one against others, on hypothetical talents such as academic aptitude. ETS called their main product, the Scholastic Aptitude Test (SAT), until even that allusion became too difficult to defend, and they reduced to calling it the SAT. As we said in Chapter 1, although for diverse groups, they provide scores that "correlate" with *some* brain function, with *some* accomplishment and with *some* potential, they do not measure intellectual function, nor accomplishment nor potential. They speak of superiority, not ability.

There are winners and losers. Equity is not intended. A few test takers get special privilege, many do not. It is easy for an unthinking world to suppose that machine scoring is neutral—not hurtful. In most places, we think, students are told or have access to their test score standing. It is easy to conclude that being told over and over, "You are inferior," is damaging.

What is the "quality of life" surrounded by people steadfast in their lowering expectations of you? Those chosen. Those not chosen.

Equity is not just a moral choice. It is a human beneficence too. Harvard College has been arguing that, without diversity, "Harvard would lose a great deal of its vitality and intellectual excellence and that the quality of the educational experience offered all students, would suffer." All students. Understanding *is* facilitated by diverse perspectives. Diversity *is* catalyst to a healthy polity. We once thought that we could promote equity by carefully measuring talent. We have, today, educational testing, a major barrier to equity.

## RANKING

In 1954, Evaluation Specialist Robert Stake (an author of this book) constructed a "quantitative aptitude" test—a test to identify incoming graduate students most likely to do well in statistical studies. He called it the Quantitative Evaluation Device (QED). It predicted well the grades in later statistics courses. It competed favorably with the Doppelt Mathematical Reasoning Test. Here is one item from the QED (see Figure 7.3).

One characteristic of such a test item is its "discrimination index." A good item contributes to the discrimination between high scorers and low scorers. It rewards high scorers and discriminates against low scorers. Stake

**Figure 7.3**

*Textbox Sample Item of the QED Test*

*Four of the five have a property.*
*Mark the one not having it.*

> (a)  *length of Joe's foot*
> (b)  *height of the tree*
> (c)  *population of Portland*
> (d)  *number of leaves on the tree*
> (e)  *final score of the game*

made a little money from graduate schools using his standardized test. But, starting to feel uncomfortable about discrimination (well, for various reasons), in about 1970 he took the test off the market. [(e) is the "right" answer. It was the choice of most high scorers.]

## COMPARING

Mandated state-wide tests are one obstacle to the caring ethic. Teacher tests are a different obstacle. Most teachers want to have tests, if only to motivate students. When they take the time, they do learn something about what students have learned. From his early research, Swedish chief educational evaluator Ulf Lundgren (1972) found that the pacing of instruction was more or less unconsciousy related to the performance of students at about the 20th percentile. When giving more attention to the very poorest performers, the better performers lose interest and learn less. It is more common for teachers to over-attend to the higher performers, thus losing the attention of (and the attention to) those toward the bottom.

Here today, we are not saying teachers should test less, but they should discriminate less, students against students. Teachers are obligated to give grades, and with big classes and with limited time, they need tests. (They could rely more on alternative assessments. They could be more supportive of nongraded schools (Louisell & Descamps, 2000)).

Is there need to discriminate among students, student against student? Do we have to compare as much as we do? A great deal of scholastic thinking involves some kinds of comparison. So too of thinking in general. We think about living, and about ethics, about caregiving, with attention to function, and problematics, and context—and often we compare with other modes of living and ethics and caregiving. We may be persuaded that it is impossible to think, without comparing (see Figure 7.4).

We spend a lot of time comparing people. And it regularly means putting people on pedestals and putting people down. We compete, partly to appear superior. We, your writers, do not suppose that we as a people could compete less, or compare less, to think less of what is superior and what is inferior. But we believe we could be less hurtful. Less hurtful.

It is not hurtful to say that Japanese cars are superior, or that American chocolate is inferior, or that Iceland is a better place to live. But it is hurtful to say that Benjamin is a slow learner. Some stereotyping is inevitable, but we need to care enough to restrain ourselves.

Every once in a while, a long while, Tomas would mention how much he liked tiramisu. Marie had never made it, but she gave it a try. Tomas said, "Well, it doesn't taste Mother's". Looking at Marie's face, he added, "But you know, I wouldn't be surprised if my tastes have changed."

**Figure 7.4**

*Said One Frog to Another, "Gosh, You're Beautiful." Said She, "Compared to What?"*

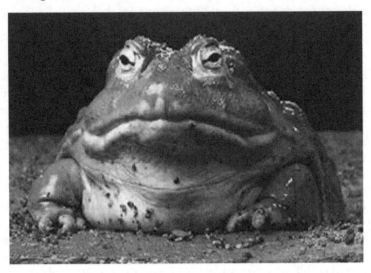

Partly because of national and state achievement standards, we compare students unnecessarily. It of little help to a youngster to know he or she was at the top again. It regularly hurts students to be shown they were wrong again and again. Almost all standardized tests are norm-referenced, they do not tell what a child has learned, only how many others made a higher number of correct answers. Grades too tell almost nothing about what a student knows.

A teacher needs to know how well a child has performed, and how well classes are progressing, but it does not help a teacher to know rankings in the class. A grade of D for Sarah should not always mean she is below Michelle who got a C. At least sometimes it should mean how good, in the eyes of the teacher, you just did.

Kids ask each other: "Wadja get?" There is an urge to know who is better and which is best. Comparison thrives in business, politics, sports and science (Moyn, 2020). And it needs to be less. But comparison burns in education. Singe-ing. Comparison of one person against others is simplistic. Especially in mandated courses, especially if the student has no choice of being there, discrimination is just plain wrong.

The *Universal Declaration of Human Rights* (2008) requires respect and protection for each and every person. Comparisons of children are seldom needed for instruction. We recognize parents' and employers' desire to know. But are not grade point averages, *rankings in class,* a violation of human rights? We can encourage teachers to support the self-respect and equity of students. We can encourage them to increase their support of a care ethic.

## The Bubble Gum Experiment

Robert Stake

On the last Friday in May, Miss Kozak announced that for the mathematics lesson, they would do research on bubble gum. She had been counting out pieces earlier and several children had strained to see what she was doing. After they returned from computer class, she quieted them down.

1:07. "Clear your desks, except for notebooks." It becomes quiet, each at his/her own place. Kozak points to five stations around the room, each with a poster identifying a bubble gum brand name and a small supply of gum.

"Okay. Just after lunch I told you we would do some research on bubble gum, drawing some graphs. What rules did I mention?" (Silence, but anticipating something good is going to happen.) "We are going to make graphs of bubble size and elasticity."

"There are different brands of bubble gum and we don't know if they are equally good at making bubbles. Each of you will make a bubble with each of five brands and, using plastic dividers, a teammate will measure the diameter." (She has placed meter sticks and calipers at each station.) "Each of you should record the measurements in your journals and on the posted sheet. Then you will take the gum, pull it into a string, and see how far you can stretch it, measuring the length with a meter stick."

"As soon as you have made both measurements, wrap that piece of gum in its wrapper and put it in the paper cup. Do not put gum anywhere except in the cup at the station. If you get it on the floor, you <u>must</u> clean it up. We don't want bubble gum on the floor or under the chairs." (Pedro claims there is gum stuck under *her* desk.) "Put the used gum in the cups."

"Listen up. Another rule is: When chewing, it's only one stick. I trust you not to take any extra. It will only works if you chew one piece. If you wad up your mouth with gum, the experiment won't work. (pause) We might have a problem if someone has a big mouth. Some people may be able to blow better than others." (laughter)

"Let's be serious about this. We don't want Mrs. Bonilla coming in and think we are goofing off. But she will understand that an experiment is important."

1:25. "We need five teams, three or four, possibly five, persons to a team. Each team is in charge of the record for one brand of gum. Is it time to break into groups? (pause) Now, divide yourselves into groups."

There is a fluttering about. Four of the more mature gather at one table; then a second group forms. Most others stay at their seats, waiting to see how things shape up. Then one by one they approach and sit down with a pair or threesome. No one approaches an existing foursome. There are now five groups of four and three kids left over, now Pedro joins the three to make a group. A couple of groups continue to reorganize, finally leaving two girls without a bubble gum station. They don't seem to mind, chatting together.

"Desks clear except for notebooks and pencils. In your journal, write the names of the people in your group. (Each person keeps their own notebook.) "Put down your own name too." Now two boys switch groups, leaving all groups but one with a single gender.

"Next, write down the names of the bubble gum, leaving space for each. Okay, do we need to know if all the gum pieces are of equal size?" (A couple of hesitant yes's.) "Let's find out and enter each size in your journal."

1. Bazooka. "How many grams in each stick, Jackie?" She reads the label: "Five grams per stick." "Write it."
2. BubbleYum. "Santiago, how much in each BubbleYum stick?" "5 grams."

(All are writing, though Manuel gets frowned down to get him started.)

3. Carefree Bubble Gum. "Jessica, how much in each stick?" "2.5 grams."
4. Bublicious. "Sandra, how much in each stick" "8 grams."
5. Extra Bubble Gum, Sugar Free. "Araceli, how big is each stick?" "2.7 grams."

"Now do your bubbles and record your results. First diameter, then elasticity. Record results at each station. (murmuring). Abraham, if you tattle, that will get you in trouble too."

1:45. All are busy chewing gum, more or less quietly. Miss Kozak reminds them they have to record other people's results, that they are doing an experiment in mathematics. Cesar gently affixes the plastic tips to measure Abraham's bubble. Touching Olivia's pink sphere, Barbara reads the angle at 32 degrees. Fatima objects, saying that the others are measuring in centimeters. Now they decide to see if Olivia can get a larger bubble.

Araceli stretches his gum to two meters but records it as 2 inches. Adolfo's pursuit of stretch threatens to get out of hand. Benny has stretched his over ten feet. It is not possible to keep the strand off the floor. Someone tells Kozak. She again says to stop tattling. "The next time I hear tattling, I'm going to ..." As to elasticity, we seem close to being in trouble. There is no place to go without crossing someone's strand. But Kozak has a smile on her face and a camera 'round her neck.

"Make sure you have recorded both length and bubble size on the paper. Time is up for your first readings. You should have both your recordings for the first piece of gum. Change stations and do it over again."

**Crisis.** Then, "Stop! Everyone, stop! The Bubblicious is all gone! It needs to be returned. Only four people had taken a piece. The box was full. Sit down. You blew it." (No pun acknowledged; Kozak is shouting in anger.)

Pointing to a stick of gum, Chunku says, "There is Bubblicious on my desk." As often the case, he is ignored. Most are still talking to each other. Kozak doesn't speak for what seems a minute. Then, "There had to be at least 10 or 15 there. I said that the only way this experiment would work if we worked as a team. If we have extra, then we can hand them out. Somebody abused this. When things get abused, they get taken away. Pedro? Anybody? I am very disappointed. This is the first time something like this has happened. Nobody is going to confess or return it?" (Silence.) "All right."

She goes out of the room, then returns. "Enough. Return to your seats. We are going to take the numbers we have and calculate the results." (Another long delay as the kids take their seats.) "Okay, we are going to add up the numbers and get the average, the mean, M-E-A-N, mean. Here they are in centimeters, write them down: 3.1, 2.6, 4.2, 3.5, 3.0, 2.9, 4.0, 3.8, 2.6, 3.5, and 3.1. Add those numbers up." (long pause.) "After you finish adding those numbers, count how many scores there are." (She counts.) "There are 11 scores. You are going to divide your total by 11." (A strained minute goes by.)

Miss Kozak bends over individuals at length, making terse comments. Some of the students seem to be struggling. Others sit quietly looking around. Kozak suggests they check their work. Now, all heads are down.

2:15. "You may want to double check it." This takes a long time. "Double check your answers." (It's as if she has just found a mistake. The decimals seem to invite mistakes.) "Be sure you have lined your numbers up right. Jose, are you done? What do you do with your total after you get it?" Pedro says, "I messed up, I believe."

It becomes apparent that Kozak does not intend to do anything with the means today. She says, "Count to yourselves. Everybody is messing each other up. Maybe if I was in a better mood, I would let you use calculators. But you messed that up too." She continues to go about the room, looking at calculations, making quiet suggestions. Chastising Abraham, she says, "First of all, you don't do math with a pen."

Then, "Abraham, go get water for the boards. There shouldn't be any talking. (pause) OK, stop what you are doing. Put your names on your worksheets. Without a sound, Santiago. Then I want everyone's attention." She is glaring at Santiago.

"What would you rather have done, the bubble gum experiment or this? Who would rather do the worksheet?" Only Pedro raises his hand. "Jessica asked me if she could use a calculator. At another time, I might have said, "Okay," but you need to be able to do this in your head. On a test you sometimes cannot use a calculator. Any comments on what happened this afternoon?" (No answer, but she waits.) Barbara says, "You are mad."

Looking around the class, "I would be a lot less mad if you had been honest. It takes a lot less to confess than to do this."

"You have two weeks of school left after today. We can go back to worksheets and reading the book. I suggest that, over the weekend, you decide whether or not we should give the class a second chance. I am really hurt. I don't go buying 16 packs of gum just to embarrass myself. Maybe I shouldn't take a chance having Ms. Bonilla come in seeing you chewing bubble gum. One thing nice about it, there were no wrappers on the floor. So, Monday we will discuss it. And maybe I will give you a second chance."

2:30. "If you want to bring it up anonymously, we can do it. You will have to prove to me that I can trust the class. As I said, this is the first time this has happened in this class. It is up to you. You may get your stuff ready to go home."

What happened during this mathematics class illustrated Miss Kozak's attachment to the children, her concern about their social development, and her desire to use the kinds of mathematics activities promoted by the school's staff development. She was nearing the end of the year and it was going to be a difficult separation for her as well as the children. She had formed personal attachment to each of them, and they for her. Hour after hour on most days went by without an expression of disrespect. Frequently she would yell, "One" then, "Two," then, "Two and a half." to get things quiet and she would sometimes stare long and hard at someone not complying with her immediate expectation, but they seldom got close to a crisis. On this day, in Kozak's eyes, they had crossed the line.

Like the high majority of teachers, new and experienced, Miss Kozak appeared here to sacrifice a good math opportunity for a social development opportunity. She could have postponed the resolution of the lost gum, carrying on the experiment with the remaining four brands. Having five brands was not critical to the activity. But it was important to her to show that trust had been breached, that theft and possibly collusion should not be treated lightly. This choice between academic learning opportunity and social ethics opportunity is not uncommon in elementary schools, but is not often discussed. It is the teacher's sense of propriety that decides, and the choice made by Miss Kozak would be supported by other teachers and parents.

She did not lose her cool. She did not seek a scapegoat. She expressed her disappointment but also her respect for the students as a whole. She did not abandon the caring ethic.

## WINNING AND LOSING

Miss Kozak recognized the attraction of competition, the arousals of competition, and made it a competition among gums rather than among children. Here she had them comparing bubble gums, not their mental abilities to measure and calculate. Mentalities were to be honed, but not exposed. Here she had safe competition. Here she had teams, and one team was to win, but not at personal cost. Some bubbles would lose, but not their blowers.

Yes, it is true, children need to learn better how to win and how to lose, both with grace. This time we saw not so much the grace of the children, but the grace of the teacher. Gracefully she bore the disappointment of her lost lesson. Gracefully she accepted the possibility of collusion. She revealed how much she cared for her lesson but cared also for the kids. Would that future lessons of the basketball court and the music hall and the junior prom could be learned as well, following the leader, taking steps toward maturity, steps toward helping others engage the caring paradigm—whether ever hearing its name.

Competition and comparing are not simple lessons. To compete and to compare can be quite easy, but to interpret their results quite difficult. To excel in one game is not once and for all. To excel in one venture is not the mark of another. A game is not a scientific sample, evidence of difference, grounds for station, justification of caste. The worth of the player remains as the worth of a person, regardless of ribbons and trophies. A caring paradigm needs be a winner in the court of human affairs.

## REFERENCES

Carse, J. P. (1986). *Finite and infinite games: A vision of life as play and possibility.* Free Press.

Cronbach, L. J., & Snow, R. E. (1977). *Aptitudes and instructional methods: A handbook for research on interactions.* Irvington.

Flanagan, J. (1960). *Overview: A history of Project Talent.* Project Talent. https://www.projecttalent.org/about/history/

Lemann, N. (2001). *The big test: The secret history of the American Meritocracy.* Farrar, Straus and Giroux.

Louisell, R., & Descamps, J. (2000). *Developing a teaching style: Methods for elementary school teachers* (2nd ed.). Waveland Press.

Lundgren, U. (1972). *Frame factors and the teaching process. A contribution to curriculum theory and theory of teaching.* Almqvist & Wiksell.

Moyn, S. (2020). *The trouble with comparisons.* The New York Review. https://www.nybooks.com/daily/2020/05/19/the-trouble-with-comparisons/

Scriven, M. (1993). *Hard won lessons program evaluation 58 (J-B PE Single Issue (Program) Evaluation).* John Wiley &Sons

Spring, J. (1988). *The sorting machine: National Educational Policy Since 1945.* Longman.

Universal Declaration of Human Rights, United Nations, General Assembly. (2008). Allen & Irwin.

# CHAPTER 8

# ABANDONMENT AND SOLIDARITY

Care seems natural but it has problems. Two problems with care are oppression and abandonment. Care ethics speaks to these problems, paying more attention to oppression than to abandonment. A child left alone, a nurse burdened, a patient bedded in a segregated room, a past friend belonging no more. Touched now, oppressed and abandoned, reduced to one. There are meta-abandonments too. Some care-giving areas are favored over others, infants over the elderly, disease over poverty. We will end this chapter with a look at the role of chance and politics and prejudice in a paradigm of care.

We so often see ourselves as individuals, thinking we are I's. But we fail to realize that the I is not prior to We (Nancy, 2000). All existence is coexistence. We are together. We are being-with, arriving alongside. This being-with is not impartial. Care keeps a tension between over-exposure to each other, and of being abandoned. Being touched by someone who cares, even the slightest touch, is something shared. For most of us, not being touched, held, affected, endangers the body. It causes hurt. Not only because we are mortal, but because we are social. We are gathered, tethered, folded together. There is no I prior to We. There were many You's before me.

## INTIMIDATION AND POLARIZATION

On television, in the newspapers, on street corners, in classrooms: there is care, there is empathy, but some of it takes false shape. Campuses, offices, walkways are scrubbed, scraped of words, ideas, and subjects that might cause offence. Sometimes we respond to even the slightest unintentional offense. It came with care, but was misreceived and misperceived. When conversationally we ask where someone comes from, it can hurt. It may be heard meaning that he or she does not belong. When we feel threatened, or feel vulnerable, we respond. We either forgive, trust and seek our own way to better the situation. Or we may appeal for help up the line, to authorities, administrative bodies, to the empowered, to whom we make the case that we feel victimized. We ask for care, but unintentionally the request polarizes; it draws darker the line of separation.

Such requests inch some people toward the precarious, the moral status of victims, although as right as they are, reporting aggression moving higher. Not unlikely, they protect themselves by closing off, creating silos, silos of isolation, and thus risking further exposure. The urge to speak out, to broadcast the accusations, grows. By doing so, they highlight their identity as precarious and predictably move away from care, from We. They emphasize their own suffering, their I. Little solution may be sought, little found. Little sense of authenticity or empowerment or care. Maybe a false sense of care: caretaking shaped to protect and intensify hurt. A false sense of safety too. They should not be blamed; they needed to protect themselves. Here, care as protection of the I, leads to moral polarization.

In times of confrontation with new viruses, new threats to health, people from distant lands get stigmatized. Some called the new coronavirus, the "China virus." Inappropriate. Demeaning. Careless. When the virus spread, the victims became fearful to admit that they had symptoms, because they might be judged or blamed. Microagression. Why not do our very best to refrain from judgment, instead to show compassion and understanding as a form of care? Here, care is about *responding* to our needs and to the needs of others. By responding and by *taking action*, we show and take *responsibility*. We do something for ourselves and others. We may offer to buy them groceries, we may bring them to the doctor, we may even advocate for them, but many times simply sitting down with them, as you know, and taking the time to listen, can be a significant act of care.

## WHO WE ARE TOGETHER

During the outbreak, many felt abandoned, lost. Doctors, nurses, and other health professionals put their lives on the line, without enough protection.

The national governments blamed cities and states, who in return blamed the national governments. While everyone wondered how to better protect nurses and doctors, what should be done for the elderly and chronically ill? Questions that arise out of solidarity. Questions that cannot be made from one circumstance only. We are connected with each other. *We are together*.

Abandonment is not just an absence of togetherness. It is a realization that those who have responsibility for the poor conditions of living in particular places are not living up to their obligations to make things better. The obligations need not be law or contract, but custom, expectation and conscience. Abandonment is the realization that a caretaker, or a community of caretakers, or a united nations of caretakers, are underperforming. The more sensitive the neglected, the greater the hurt—and the greater the irresponsibility. Do the caretakers respond by desensitizing the neglected, or by working to game the system, the priorities of need, the checks and balances, so there becomes less by which to be offended? Equity is not achieved by raising the blindness to inequity.

## An Immigrant Child

Brinda Jegatheesan (2019)

With her 7-year old daughter Carlotta, Yolanda came to the United States as an undocumented worker to find employment. Carlotta's father Pedro remained on his family's property in Mexico. As an undocumented immigrant Yolanda had restrictions on leaving the U.S. Four months a year, during the summer and winter school holidays, Carlotta returned to Mexico to spend time with her father and paternal grandparents and her beloved pet chicken, Chuck E. Cheese, all of whom lived on Pedro's farm. By age seven Carlotta had begun to experience the physical and psychological pains of the separations from her parents, grandparents and her pet chicken.

Although Carlotta only spent summer and winter holidays with Chuck E. Cheese in Mexico, she was very attached to him. Carlotta often talked about how happy she was when she was with her pet and how much she missed Chuck E. Cheese each time she returned to the states. She explained that she could not have a pet in the U.S. because of their living arrangements. Her parents and extended family members in the U.S. and Mexico recognized her bond with the chicken and worked hard to ensure that she received emotional support during her time away from her pet. They provided her with a range of cross-border communication channels (e.g., phone calls, mailing of photographs of her pet and gifts) to continue Carlotta's close relationship with her chicken. For example, Yolanda ensured that her daughter's birthdays were traditionally celebrated in the U.S. with the much anticipated festivities held at the local Chuck E. Cheese pizzeria and arcade; whereas her pet Chuck E. Cheese' birthdays were celebrated in Mexico with her father and grandparents helping to facilitate the celebrations. Photographs were shared back and forth between family members, including frequent phone from relatives in Mexico to inform Carlotta about how well her chicken was doing and was waiting for her to visit during her summer break.

We cannot expect that others should take responsibility for situations for which we together are responsible. Who decides who needs most the last pack of toilet paper? Instead of hoarding toilet paper, every one of us is called to care about the others by not buying all available goods. Ideally, we practice *solidarity*. We *trust*. We treat people fully as ones of us. According to Joan Tronto (2013) the three pillars of a caring society are: solidarity, equality, and trust. Share products with those who need them the most, trust that we will have enough for ourselves. In times when there are no clear-cut ethical guidelines to follow, the situation is too threatening for general rules. Soon, many stores put limits on products to be bought. No more than three hand sanitizers. But what if someone suffers from a chronic illness and is more vulnerable to infection than others? Should people without a chronic illness share their packages? Reaching decisions on the best path to follow, there is a need to take subtle differences, situations, into consideration. Trust the pharmacist. Trust the receptionist.

## SOLIDARITY

According to some, solidarity is at the root of the ethical. Solidarity is an awareness, subjective, incalculable. According to political scientist Bruce Jennings, "It produces the response for ethical action in the presence of an-other in peril—another who is a moral subject, a being with a visage, a gaze, an ontological claim to stake, a political inheritance to claim, a place of membership rightfully to occupy" (Jennings, 2018, p. 3). Solidarity can be personal, communal and political. Personal, it refers to bonds of loyalty, togetherness, because of our affiliations. We mentioned this back in the first chapter, and will get back to it in the last. Affiliations determine what we do for each other. Solidarity can also be communal and political: it becomes instrumental and strategic for survival, rather than an existential way of being, something that we hold dear, just because it matters to us. Jodi Dean wrote about conventional and reflective solidarity (Dean, 1996). Bruce Jennings (2018) spoke of solidarity as a moral trajectory, an image that became real during the crisis of the new coronavirus.

For Tomas and Marie, what did the covid-19 lock-down feel like? Was it more like *abandonment* or more like *solidarity*? They had wanted to feel a part of the neighborhood, and world effort, to keep people safe. But before it was over, they had strong feelings of being *abandoned*.

## CARING CITIZENS

On national and international levels we were expected to be "pandemic citizens" (Maunula, 2013, p. 14). We were called to follow regulations by being rational, responsible citizens. It was urged that we act in the interest of the collective. Compliance, self-mastery, self-protection, and caring are aligned with that view. But this vital view is challenging too, because people are imagined to be capable of compliance and self-mastery. The reality is different. People are capable, and vulnerable too. They cannot "self-master" their lives all the time and in many situations. Some of us carry particular responsibilities that conflict with these expectations. For example, the careworker who is exhausted but who carries on because nobody else is able to stand in. Who takes care of her? Just as some citizens have gone crazy with gun violence, and just as some attempt to buy companies for exclusive rights on vaccines, we could not predict how others will respond to the virus, nor could we predict how the virus will develop in the future. We cannot ask the virus. It too does not know. From a care perspective, we are open to learning about how to relate to uncertainty and abandonment.

A caring citizen, in line with Joan Tronto's work on the *homines curans* (Tronto, 2017) (caring people), demands for us to see human beings as being closely interconnected with others in webs of care. Others, as in other human beings, but also as in non-human others. Some of those others are more vulnerable and precarious. Yes: as a pandemic citizen, social distancing has been crucial. As a caring citizen, we also search for ways to stay connected with close and distant others. To keep social distancing healthy, we need an outlook on how to support people who are living in isolation. How they can preserve and maintain their relationships, while complying with regulations. For many, being in isolation, at least for a while, may come with the gift of time, silence and solitude. But what if some do not experience this gift at all? What if our jobs are on the line? What if we miss graduation day? What if we lose that which makes us human: the experience of being close to someone or someplace we care about?

The pandemic called and still calls for global solidarity. An entwined solidarity that assists us in responding to what is unraveling in and around us. A solidarity that is not restricted to us as humans, but that respects our entanglements with matter and a world of living creatures. But first, let us take a close-up but far-distant look at solidarity. Here is a scene from the south of China. Like stories in other chapters, we are reminded of how caring reaches people and of how important it is (is it not for everyone?) to have a caring surround.

## Seeking Life Betterment: An Informal Spiritual/Religion Group of Old Rural Women in Zhejiang, China

Yali Feng (n.d.), *University of Illinois*

If you walk along one coastline of Southern rural China, you come across an ordinary room whose three windows face east, south, and north, emanating an almost inaudible but rhythmic chant and periodic laughter. You might feel a magic power, peaceful and soothing. You cannot help but look in the window. Eight old women, ages 60 to 80, sit 'round a table. Their dresses are neat and their expression mild. Each holds a pile of small yellow papers, a half-inch wide, two inches long. At intervals they flip up a piece of paper. If you ask them, they will tell you they are chanting sutra and counting with the papers, one piece for each chant.

At the center of the table stands a burning stick of incense; around it, some pastry and fruits. Most of the space on the table is occupied by those yellow papers. Other tables line the walls holding paper-made stuff, such as gold ingots (typical symbol for wealth in China culture), colorful lotuses made from wax paper, and paper-cut patterns (symbols for longevity, wealth, luck, and so on). If you stay long enough, you find this scenario can last for roughly from 6:30 A.M. to 10:30 A.M. and 12:00 P.M. to 4:00 P.M. for up to 8 days. If you roam further in southern rural China, you will come across others, none of them described in media, just women in a sutra-chanting group.

**Growing Old.** Aging is a world-wide issue, and so in China, which in 2006 had over 150 million people aged 60 years and over, which is roughly 21% of the world's elderly population. Of those, 108 million lived in rural areas. As females live longer than males, they comprise a larger part of that population. So far, there is little, if any, welfare or public support for these women. They are not a topic of Chinese policy.

From the Buddhist view point, this chanting appears of little value to the women, possibly even being harmful to their spiritual health. However, we should understand the chanting in its life context. Due to their poor economic, educational, and physical status, old rural women actually have been excluded from mainstream society, deprived of sharing the fruits of social and economic development. They do not know Mandarin and media such as TV mean little to them. What they can do, and what they do most besides housework, is chanting simple sutra. The importance of sutra chanting is self-evident. If one thinks of these activities as fulfilling, it is a meaningful role for these women.

**This Setting.** In 2008 Orange Village had 278 households with a population of about 900. The average yearly income was about 4,000 RMB, i.e.,

$547, per capita. The village lies on the coastline in Ningbo District in Zhejiang Province, in southeastern China. Ningbo is a famous port city with a 7,000-year history. It was one of the earliest cities opened to the West. Zhejiang is among the richest provinces. The village is 1.5 hours from Ningbo, 4 hours north of Shanghai.

Hundreds of years ago, the village, just as other villages nearby, was ocean. Today we can still see the furrows left behind by the powerful sea. The main road for the village was once a sea bank built by ancestors. Today you can get seafood by bike in 20 minutes. The villagers who were fishermen are now farmers.

Just like most of the forerunners who actively claimed land from the sea, their descendants remain diligent and active in earning a living. They enjoy an unpressured life, as seen at the two local grocery stores, the entertainment and information centers, where villagers spend leisure time playing Mahjong and cards and exchanging news, information, and gossip. If one wants to know the unemployment situation in Chinese rural area, you can get first-hand information by observing the grocery stores. Almost all of the agriculture activities here are still handled by hand, just as thousands of years ago, but herbicide, pesticide and fertilizer save time and labor. Orange Village has advantages that contribute to its agriculture. First, it is close to the national economic center of Shanghai. Selling is not a problem despite dramatically fluctuating prices. Second, there is a large irrigation facility for droughts and for draining flood water. Crop production is stable when the weather is not terribly bad.

Nearly every villager grows rice for their own food and mandarin oranges as a main income. Every household has orange trees, from several dozen to several hundred. An average tree can produce 20 to 100 RMB each year. Some grow a little cotton, wheat, soybeans, horse beans, watermelon, or corn to earn side money. Most of the young men in Orange Village work a while in big cities such as Beijing and Shanghai as migrant workers. But few of them have settled there. Between 2000 and 2010 many returned because several big factories making office supplies were built nearby, hiring thousands.

Though there are several options for the young people to earn money, the choice for the old is slim. They lead a traditional life. Some are too old to take care of orange trees and field work, and so they rent their land to other villagers. The rent differs every year according to the orange prices. It was 5 RMB for each tree for several years, and then it became 20 RMB (0.8 RMB for 500g, that is about ten cents a pound). As the orange price was especially bad in 2007-2008 (0.3 RMB for 500g), rents plunged in 2008. Fields have been allotted to every family by the government since 1979. The rent for every mu (Chinese unit of area, 1/15 of a hectare) is about 200 RMB, plus a small amount of what is produced.

No public income, food, or housing support is provided by the government. Rural elders depend on their own labor, orange trees and field rent, and support from children. Some of the aged are so good at playing mahjong that they can win enough money to support themselves.

**The People.** In daily life, the elders get help from neighbors as well as from their children. Orange Village is a close-knit, typical Chinese rural community. Except for youth who leave for higher education, everyone knows each other. Age hierarchy and respect for authority have their expression in daily detail. Being born here and dying here, villagers know the importance of respecting the aged and giving support when in need. Everyone knows they will have their turn. Neighbors and village leaders get involved in mediation if there are serious family conflicts. Their sons-in-law and daughters-in-law might not always show filial piety,[1] but neighbors are usually nice to each other. On occasion, the widowed elders will be given food by neighbors, such as zhongzi on Dragon Boat Festival Day, sweet dumpling on Lantern day, tree rice cake on April 8, and so on. In crises, they provide substantial support, from emotional help to finance. Of course, reciprocation is expected. For older females it varies, for most have lived with a husband's family.

Most of the aged in the village are illiterate, but understand a little Mandarin. They often watch some TV in bed before sleeping. But the most important leisure activity is playing mahjong at the grocery stores. Those who are too poor to play sit beside the mahjong table and chat.

The children go to primary and secondary school in a small town 3.5 km away. It is rare to see them in the daytime. A few old women hold the responsibility of taking care of infants and toddlers when their parents work at sites far from the village.

Connected to a temple, each charting group consists of eight women with an age total set firmly at 500 years. Most of the old women are primary housekeepers, and usually are the only one in a household responsible for housework. When they have time, they go out to chat with each other. Coming to Orange Village, every visitor receives a warm welcome no matter how often they visit and how close they live. The hostess boils water and makes a cup of green tea and takes out snacks saved for such occasions. This courtesy is deeply established. On special occasions, they visit a nearby temple to burn incense (a ritual offering) together, occasions including: the birthday of Laoye (the local god who protects the local people), i.e., August 16 in the Chinese calendar, and the first morning of the Chinese New Year.

**The Author.** I was born and raised in Orange village. I obtained entry into a group as a daughter of a member and a daughter of the neighborhood. I have been participating in their life, in this way or that, for very long with the knowledge about sutra chanting and this particular group coming slowly.

As a young woman around 30, I am not one of the members, but over time I have been their friend and supporter. My maternal grandma was Buddhist and practiced chanting daily. When I was 3 or 4 years old, I was sent to live with her, because my family did not have enough food and another sister was going to be born. Unintelligible chanting and faded memories are outlined by exciting candies. She would give me coins to buy candies while she chanted and when I deliberately whined at how lonely I was.

Seventeen years later, my Mom learned Heart Sutra when she broke her leg and could not work on the farm. Since then, she has increasingly attended sutra chanting. On holidays, I escorted her to their gathering place and chatted with the members. Sometimes I brought snacks. When it rained, I took some umbrellas for them. I called and asked their situation when I was in universities far from the village. I know every one of them very well.

In July 2006, I went back home and lived with my Mom. I helped her prepare items for the sutra chant, such as the paper-cuts and paper gold ingots. I was there listening when she dropped around the village for casual chats. Gradually, I became interested in this sutra chanting group and was intrigued by its meaning in their life. Mom did not understand why I was interested in "such trivial and daily" things, but was supportive and told her group. A few days later, they asked me curiously why I would be interested in such unimportant things. That started my interviews. They ended around November 2007 when I returned to the U.S. In June 2008, I went back to China. I still keep contact with the participants through phone calls.

**Sutra Chanting.** By rule, the total age (Chinese lunar age) of the eight female participants must be exactly 500 years. Here they ranged from 54 to 71. Four were illiterate. Pao and Shan did recognize some words. Chuan was the only one who could read a little. None of them spoke Mandarin. Everyone had stories of sickness, a condition often triggering the start of sutra chanting and later to joining a chanting group.

The women spent most of their days in housework and taking care of grandchildren, but some also worked in the field in midseason. Sometimes, they got financial support from their kids. They were poor, but if not in an accident or sickness, they made ends meet. They watched for work opportunity that did not demand high physical requirement.

Sutra chanting is practiced widely and naturally in China, and it is taken for granted that it will become a life style for women when they reach a certain age. I asked them, "Would you please tell me when you began to chant with the 500-year sutra? Why did you join the group? Or what made you start?" The answers were similar and repeated over and over again, "My body wore out. Everyone [in my family] is working [in field]. I can't. All I can do is chanting sutra. What else is there to do?"

**Conversations.** The women talk at breaks and during chanting, village news, what they cared most about in their lives: aging (especially accidents and health problem caused by aging), death, family and marriage. They share feelings, joke about themselves. My Mom complains, "I used to work outside in the fields, raised six kids. Work, work, work, every day. Didn't feel a thing. Now, I always feel exhausted. I am useless and dependent. I can only do some housework. My back hurts so much that I could not stand when I washed the sheets yesterday." Others tell what happened to them yesterday, reminding them of their aging, sometimes, sharing medical information.

They talk about how they prefer to die, especially now after the death of Qing and Jane. Qing was a member of a 500-year sutra-chanting group for one year and Jane had been earlier. Qing was very independent, died from liver cancer. She suffered long periods of pain before she told anyone and was still working the day before she died. Quite to the contrary, Jane was very dependent. After a stroke, she refused to exercise although she still could walk in the house without help. She cried aloud whenever there was anyone to hear, whining about her misfortune and maltreatment from sons and daughters-in-law. Gradually, neighbors avoided her. She had two sons living in the same house, and one son, one daughter, and one brother nearby, but felt deserted. From their talking, it seems the members admired Qing and were afraid of Jane. They did not want to end their lives in Jane's condition.

The women learned from the problems that arose from deaths and funerals of neighbors. They pushed each other to prepare for their own funeral, "The more you prepare now, the less trouble you will bring to your children." "Prepare earlier before you get too old. Xiu's Mom (Xiu is a neighbor) used to talk about her dying several years ago. Look at her now. She is very sick and totally avoids the topic." "If you prepare for yourself now, you can choose the clothes to wear when you die." Most of them had prepared their grave clothes, and sutra packages to be burned at the funeral.

Family and marriage issues are a common topic, either their own or others'. Shan had problems with her daughter-in-law and wept a lot during chant talking. She did not know how to improve the relationship. The members made suggestions.

My Mom would tell us village news when she came back from group activity—A's wife ran away, B's child bought furniture for her parents, C's pig had babies, D fertilized his orange trees, the soybean price dropped, and on.

Sometimes the news was international. Once Mom told me the orange price in our village was low because the U.S. was fighting with Iraq. She explained: the price was low because there are fewer buyers in North China, which is because diesel oil was in short supply and orange delivery became a big problem. I was very surprised.

Pao had come home after spending two months in Zhoushan, where her son lives, to take care of her grandson. Late one evening, after dinner, we were at Chuan's home. Pao came in with a smile on her face. Everyone in the room screamed, so glad to see her. We asked how she was doing.

Pao exhaled a long breath and said, "Finally, I came back," tears in her eyes. "Food was good, place is nice, not too much housework to do, not tiring at all. I was glad to be with my son and his family. But I was just not happy. I almost died because my heart was toasting in the loneliness. When my grandson went to school, son and daughter-in-law went to work, and I was all alone. I did not know what to do. I cried. I had to cover my crying …"

My Mom added, "Otherwise, your son would be annoyed and think you ungrateful and unappreciative, saying: "We did not abuse you. Treated you with respect. Gave you money. Bought you nice food …" I had heard it before. My sister often invited my Mom to stay with them in the county. But Mom was reluctant. She would start packing to go home the first day she got there.

"Exactly," said Pao, "I did not have any reason to be unhappy there. My son does not understand. Neither do I. But I just could not control myself." Tears again came to her eyes. Chuan said, "Golden house, silver house, none can compare with my own decrepit house." Everybody nodded, looking with empathy at Pao. Pao continued, "I did not know I would miss you guys so much. The time there was like prison. I am so glad I am back. But my son wants me there when my grandson ... "

Chuan asked, "Why didn't you go around and spend time with the neighbors?" Pao said, "I was afraid of getting lost, which would bring trouble to my son. And, it is no fun to go out. I do not understand their dialect." One's resources and social supports often are taken for granted, but realized when taken away. When Pao and my Mom visited their children, they were no longer in touch with their sutra group members.

Pao's story suggests that the group's powerful emotional support reduced anxiety, helplessness, depression, and loneliness during aging. The function of the group might be understood better when we consider the uniqueness of aging. Unlike the teenage period, in which struggles and embarrassment can be successfully put aside by most people because they know there is a future, aging is different. It waits for everyone ahead and cannot be imagined until it starts. But once it starts, it will always be with you to the last breath, like a shadow that follows your body. The most terrible thing is that its process really can only be understood well by those who are experiencing it. The chanting group promotes psychological well-being and positive togetherness of these old women through expressing, recognizing, sharing, and releasing the feeling of role loss in the family and the frustrating experience of aging.

## SUSPICION AND STANDING UP

Our world's societies neither recognize nor acknowledge Pao's economic worth. For society, she no longer counts, she is just a burden. She's worthless. What if society would use its robust accounting skills to record her worth? What if we cared as much about measuring "care worth" as we do about property worth? Here, "worth" is practicing solidarity. Solidarity means *standing up* for people who are more vulnerable than others, whose contribution and place are not immediately visible, but worth (in our advanced perception) as much as those of others. Solidarity means not being suspicious when you, as an advisor, visit a client for a conversation.

We do not imply that there should be no scrutiny, no critical examination. It is something to work on.

We would promote a solidarity that advocates, defends, pleads the cause of the other (Jennings, 2018, p. 5). One that stands up against exclusion and abandonment. Stands up against the implementation of norms and criteria that fail to take situations and contexts into consideration. You as reader and we as writers can promote a solidarity that translates norms to the particular lives that are at stake. A solidarity that *stands up with* the other. Putting ourselves next to another, empathizing, understanding their lifeworld as much as possible. Moral solidarity is about *engaging* with the other, equal as can be, with respect and dignity, in a reciprocal way. Equitable. Moral recognition is rare, but necessary for unlocking more of the potential of others and their others and their others.

## SOLITUDE AND SILENCE

Solidarity asks for engagement and attachment with others. On the other side of the continuum, there is detachment, solitude, and individualism. Virginia Woolf was curious about this: "If as novelist you wish to test man in all his relationships, the proper antagonist is man; his ordeal is in society, not solitude" (Woolf, 1932, p. 259). We need solitude and silence, however, to care properly, to be into togetherness properly. In silence and solitude, we can connect with ourselves: with our longings, emotions, thoughts, dark and lighter sides. We need that conscious "I" to be well with others. To do well. A togetherness that is without the "I" would not be a "productive" togetherness. It would be a fusion, not a real encounter with others. When we care for ourselves, we are caring for the self as polyphonic (Leget, 2017). Our polyphony contains emotional, physical, sociocultural, political, existential, and spiritual voices. We need silence and solitude to hear those voices, to reflect, reconnect with ourselves. But not all silence and solitude work like that. Some silences and solitudes foster reflection, while others do not. A silence that feels uncomfortable, alone and lonely, can abandon us to misery and self-pity. A silence that feels rich, deepening and nourishing can lift us up. Silence and solitude can have many faces. They are rare commodities. Thus, in silence and solitude, we experience our inner life that is about togetherness too. A togetherness with ourselves. It is about care for ourselves and our inner world. One care ethicist, Carlo Leget, captured this concept as inner space (Leget, 2017). Inner space, as a quality of our awareness that is present in every day phenomena like friendliness, politeness, and humor, and is a necessary condition of attentive listening, good conversations and encounters. Cultivating an inner space we may better deal with contrary voices. It may be easier to find the right balance between care for ourselves, and care for others.

## REFERENCES

Dean, J. (1996). *Solidarity of strangers*. University of California Press.

Feng, Y. (n.d.). *Seeking life betterment: An informal spiritual/religion group of old rural women in Zhejiang, China* (Unpublished doctoral dissertation). Urbana, University of Illinois.

Jegatheesan, B. (2019). Influence of cultural and religious factor o attitudes toward animals. In A. Fine (Ed.), *Handbook on animal-assisted therapy*. Elsevier. https://dol.org/10.1016/B978-0-12-815395-6.00004-3

Jennings, B. (2018). Solidarity and care as relational practices. *Bioethics, 32*(9), 553–561. https://dol.org/10.1111/bioe.12510

Leget, C. (2017). *Art of living, art of dying: Spiritual care for a good death*. Jessica Kingsley Publishers.

Maunula, L. (2013). The pandemic subject: Canadian pandemic plans and communicating with the public about an influenza pandemic. *Health Policy, 9*(SP), 14–25.

Nancy, J. L. (2000). *Being singular plural*. Stanford University Press.

Tronto, J. (2017). There is an alternative: Homines curans and the limits of neoliberalism. *International Journal of Care and Caring, 1*(1), 27–43.

Tronto, J. (2013). *Caring democracy: Markets, equality and justice*. New York University Press.

Woolf, V. (1932). How should one read a book? In A. McNeillie (Ed.), *The common reader* (p. 259). Hartcourt.

## NOTE

1. Simply speaking, filial piety means children do what their parents want and act not against their parents' will. For the adults, filial piety means they support their parents' lives financially.

# CHAPTER 9

# NATURE AND
# THE HUMANITIES

Caring for people and caring for nature can be treated as separate responsibilities but we treat them both in this book as vital parts of a care paradigm. The methods and the immediacies may be different, but they are bonded as commitments. If in ways we fail either, the other will suffer. As of this writing, we have put almost eight billion people on this earth. Even in their most generous and caring moments, these billions take more than they give. Even the oceans are landfill. We do not have the means, it seems, nor the will, to save either the human condition or the earth beneath and above. But it is within our power to slow the assault. We have at times shown we can be heroic.

Consider the words of Chief Joseph of the Nez Perce, one of the greatest of Indian leaders. His people were repeatedly promised their Western lands, then displaced repeatedly, finally forcibly settled on Oklahoma reservations. He spoke eloquently to a session of Congress, but his tribe was not returned to their home. These were his opening lines.

> My friends, I have been asked to show you my heart. I am glad to have a chance to do so. I want the white people to understand my people
>
> Some of you think an Indian is like a wild animal. This is a great mistake. I will tell you all about our people, and then you can judge whether an Indian is a man or not.
>
> I believe much trouble would be saved if we opened our hearts more. I will tell you in my way how the Indian sees things. The white man has more

*a Paradigm of Care,* pp. 107–121

words to tell. You know how they look to him, but it does not require many words to speak the truth.

What I have to say will come straight from my heart, and I will speak with a straight tongue. The Great Spirit is looking at me, and will hear me.

The earth is the mother of all people, and all people should have equal rights upon it. (Speech by Chief Joseph, 1879)

## THE GOOD EARTH

Our planet is one of us, and it is vulnerable. With vulnerability comes the constant possibility of harm (Fineman, 2008). Vulnerability cannot be ignored or shoved under the carpet. Where there is life, there is exposure. We humans are vulnerable, but animals, plants, trees, the climate, and other things, too, are disposed to harm and hurt. We can be socially hurt, bodily and emotionally. We can be left alone, lose jobs, and lose possessions. We can be attacked, discriminated, humiliated or disrespected. To not get hurt we protect ourselves. We protect our children, our belongings, our beliefs, and our habits. We protect by closing off, exercising control, by stepping out of relations, by leaving situations. Sometimes successfully, many times causing more harm and hurt. But meanwhile, no matter how keen or thoughtless our self-protection, we take other things for granted. Many things. We forget to protect some of which is vital to our lives and to living: the air that we need to fill our lungs, the trees that hold together the ground underneath our feet, the water that surrounds our lands.

Anyone who lives well off the equator has noticed how the boundaries of the seasons blur. They say that insects and birds predict the weather. They say that they sense the seasons better than we do. But it hurts to see them starting their nests a couple of days before a snowstorm. It hurts to hear of disoriented whales, flailing on the beach. Our earth is perplexed, it is subject to a force that we all know too well, a force called: the human.

Today, per second, 20 football fields of forests disappear. These trees turn into paper or into pulp. They end up in grocery stores as packaging, or advertisements in mailboxes, thrown away without a look. That is 20 times 60 trees an hour. Tree cutting is a multi-billion-dollar industry attacking forests worldwide—temporarily. We will not live to see replacements. Tree slaughter not only hurts forests, but local communities and wildlife too.

With vulnerability comes dependency. We are dependent on trees, and trees depend on us. They clear our air. They absorb smells and dangerous gases. Their leaves and basts work hard to exhale the oxygen that we need so badly. Some folks believe we can talk to trees, that they have a soul, that they radiate cosmic tenderness (Denver, 2014). We do not know, but we do see that a forest heals its creatures. Trees purify our hearts and minds.

Despite our dependency on trees, only some of us notice them, let alone care for them. Only some of us pay attention to their welfare. Only some of us are willing to notice the canopy, or the weed trees by the tracks. They belong too. Our dependency is nested: we are not alone; we are part of a chain, a biosphere. As a child, we were taken care of by our mother. Our mother had a friend. The friend needed another friend. We all rely upon a chain of others, sometimes the link familiar, sometimes a complete stranger. Our bonds are vital for living our lives as well as possible.

But a tree, no matter how old or young, or beautiful or ugly, a tree stands out there, deeply rooted, often alone and half-time naked, in the great wide open. It can be surrounded by other trees, but those cannot jump in the way to prevent its mate from being cut and hurt and used for human "necessities." Isolation from our trees, is one of the biggest mistakes of modern humankind. We take pride in our intellect, in our multi-billion-dollar industries. But we take too little pride in our resources, stripping them of strength and power. We focus on national growth but much of it is national devastation. We need to acknowledge once again, that in the end, the human mind is bent toward destruction. Vulnerable to pride and greed. Digging its own grave. There are good protections, and bad ones. There is good care with bad consequences, and there is bad care with good endings. Tree care has become bad and bad.

Nature could be less vulnerable to hurt and exploitation were we to consider other points of view. It might begin with us counting the annual rings. Some trees grow older than humans will ever be. The oldest tree is circumscribed at 4,800 years. And although numbers tell little of quality, and although we cannot compare trees with humans, we can respect the tree as a living entity. Take how the Maori of New Zealand treat their land and earthhood. By political recalculation, their Whanganui River and Te Urewera Forest have legal personhood. Is this a talisman? It may illustrate the evolving relationships with nonhuman nature.

Newly acknowledging the river and the forest takes note of colonial history and past exploitation of ecological resources. Now, the river and the forest can own "themselves." They should no longer be owned or oppressed by others. Before this was possible, another acknowledgement was attained: the plurality of ontologies existing next to each other (Fitzgerald, 2019). The Maori people viewed relationships between humans and (nonhuman) nature differently from the people arriving from the West. According to the Maori, humans are entangled with nature, codependent. Nature is not there for humans to "use." They are not separated from it, should not, merely by anthropocentric logic, control it. The care ethics scholar Maggie Fitzgerald (2019) wrote about this:

This case, I suggest, is an example of a conflict between two worlds. On the one hand, the New Zealand Government—constituted by the modern world—constructs and understands the Whanganui River as property. On the other hand, the Māori tribe of Whanganui understands the river as an ancestor and still-living kin. However, under the partition of the perceptible, inherent to modernity, the Māori world was rendered unintelligible for over 140 years; the Whanganui River was not viewed by the State as kin, or as a living entity, but rather was treated as property. Indeed, even the Māori's own view of/relationship with the river as kin was not acknowledged by the State. As a result, the reproduction of the Māori people's world was made precarious, as the river was both treated in a way that violated the logic of their world and denied a subject status that was key to their broader ontological and epistemological framework. (p. 9)

The 140-year struggle to recognize the Whanganui River as a living entity, then, is an example of politics as defined by Rancière. In this case, the Māori fought to bring into relationship two incommensurable logics: their own understanding of the river as kin and the view of nature as property that in part constitutes modernity. In so doing, they made visible that which was invisible, namely, their relationship with the Whanganui River and the world of which this relationship is a part. Importantly, in bringing together these two incommensurable logics, equivocation is not achieved. The Government of New Zealand does not see the river as a human, nor do the Māori fully embody the legal framework which facilitated this recognition. Rather, in bringing together these two logics, a tentative reconfiguration of the partition of the perceptible is achieved, in which "the contradiction of two worlds in a single world" is foregrounded. (Rancière, 1999, p. 27)

Last year, in Toledo, Ohio, people voted to grant legal standing to Lake Erie, a juridical protection. Of course, we need more substantial forms of protection, forms that express our common care. Next to the gaze of homage, we need justice too. We need to rationally recognize what is ethically right. We need regulations and evaluations of what is good and what is bad. Rules to apply impartially to decisions about how we treat the world, how to tame greed and pride. We slowly start to accept that we need protection from ourselves. That we need to let go of self-importance and decenter our desires. For us to succumb to this, for us to be wholly unpretentious and modest, may be among the hardest things to do. Care for modesty and humility could form the roots of a healthy ecosystem. All parts of that system have a vulnerable body, made from limbs and muscles, rings, and basts. All parts of the system depend as much on the attachments as on the air that surrounds them. If only we could more strongly feel this intimacy.

In 1962, Rachel Carson published *Silent Spring*, detailing effects on the environment caused by indiscriminate use of pesticides. Author Barbara Kingsolver (2002, ) used the issue to vivify the tensions among rural neighbors in her novel, *Prodigal Summer*. Here is part of her dialogue between two Appalachian farmers, Nannie Rawley and Garnett Walker, both seeing themselves caretakers of nature, separately their apple and hickory trees.

## An Excerpt From *Prodigal Summer*

Barbara Kingsolver

... and scooted her bushel forward so they faced each other directly, within spitting distance. "What we need is to have a good, levelheaded talk about this pesticide business, farmer to farmer."

"... It's the middle of July, he said. "The caterpillars are on my seedling like the plague. If I didn't spray, I'd lose all this year's new crosses."

"See, but you're killing all my beneficials. You're killing my pollinators. You're killing the songbirds that eat the bugs. You're just a regular death angel, Mr. Walker."

"I have to take care of my chestnuts," he replied firmly.

She gave him a hard look. "Mr. Walker, is it my imagination, or do you really think your chestnuts are more important than my apples? Just because you're a man and I'm a woman? You seem to forget, my apple crop is my living. Your trees are a *hobby*."

Now, that was low. Garnett should have called on the phone. Talking to a brainless machine would beat this. "I never said a thing about your apples. I'm helping you out by spraying. The caterpillars would be over here next."

"They *are* over here. I can keep them under control my own way, normally. But your spraying always causes a caterpillar boom."

He shook his head. "How many times do I have to listen to that nonsense?"

She leaned forward, her eyes growing wide. "Until you've *heard* it!"

"I've heard it. Too many times."

"No, now, I haven't explained it to you right. I always had a hunch, but I couldn't put it in words. And, see, last month they had a piece on it in the *Orchardman's Journal*. It's a whole scientific thing, a principle. Do you want me to get you the magazine, or just explain it in my own words?"

"I don't think I have any choice," he said. "I'll listen for the flaw in your reasoning. Then you'll have to hush up about this for good."

"Good," she said, shifting her bottom on the basket. "All right, now. Goodness, I feel a little bit nervous. Like I'm back in college, taking an exam." The anxious way she looked up at him reminded Garnett of all the years of boys who'd feared him in his vo-ag classes. He wasn't a mean teacher; he'd just insisted that they get things *right*. Yet they'd dreaded him for it. They were never his chums, as they were with Con Ricketts in shop, for instance. It made for a long, lonely life, this business of getting things right.

"Okay, here we go," she said finally, clasping her hands together. "There are two main kind of bugs, your plant eaters and your bug eaters."

"That's right," he said patiently. "Aphids, Japanese beetles, and caterpillars all eat plants. To name just a few. Ladybugs eat other small bugs."

"Ladybugs do," she agreed. "Also, spiders, hornets, cicada killers, and a bunch of other wasps, plus your sawflies and parasitic hymenoptera, and lots more. So out in your field you have predators and herbivores. You with me so far?"

He waved a hand in the air. "I taught vocational agriculture for half as long as you've been alive. You have to get up early in the morning to surprise an old man like me." Although, truth to tell, Garnett had never heard of parasitic hymenoptera.

"Well, all right. Your herbivores have certain characteristics."

"They eat plants."

"Yes. You'd call them pests. And they reproduce fast."

"Don't I know it!" Garnett declared.

"Predator bugs don't reproduce so fast, as a rule. But see, that works out right in nature because one predator eats a world of pest bugs in its life. The plant eaters have to go faster just to hold their ground. They're in balance with each other. So far, so good?"

Garnett nodded. He found himself listening more carefully than he'd expected.

"All right. When you spray a field with a broad-spectrum insecticide like Sevin, you kill pest bugs and the predator bugs, bang. If the predators and prey are balanced out to start with, and they both get knocked back the same amount, then the pests that survive will *increase* after the spraying, fast, because most of their enemies have just disappeared. And the predators will *decrease* because they've lost most of their food supply. So in the lag between sprayings, you end up boosting the number of the bugs you don't want and wiping out the ones you need. And every time you spray, it gets worse."

"And then?" Garnett asked, concentrating on this.

She looked at him. "And that's it. I'm done. The Volterra principle."

Garnett felt hoodwinked. How could she do this every time? In another day and age they'd have burned her for a witch. (Kingsolver, 2002, pp. 273–275)

## CLIMATE CHANGE

One biggest challenge is care for our climate. We can care because of economic reasons or because we feel socially pressured, but perhaps it would ideally spark from a sense of urgency for all the living things in our environment. On March 31, 2020, Barack Obama tweeted: "We've seen all too terribly the consequences of those who denied warnings of a pandemic. We can't afford any more consequences of climate denial. All of us, especially young people, have to demand better of our government at every level and vote this fall" (Obama, 2020). This was a call in response to weakened fuel economy standards, the U.S. leaving the Paris Agreement, and many other ignored or rejected climate actions. Some argue that denying climate change is denying our human vulnerability and the vulnerability of the earth. Just as with covid-19, the severity of the climate crisis can overwhelm people to such an extent that they "disconnect," freeze, become numb. Not because they don't care, but because they are *incapable* of this kind of caring. The severity of the situation is too much to handle.

The Dutch care ethicist Henk Manschot speaks of a "contrast experience" (Manschot, 2016, p. 10) showing us that critical experiences like hurricanes, tsunami's, wildfires, or other grand climate events disrupt our everyday lives in practical ways, but also touch us in an existential way. Manschot (2016) learns from the philosopher Nietzsche, who argued that the "earth is ill, and the illness is called the human being" (p. 12). The remedy, according to Nietzsche was: to remain faithful to the earth. To do this, he believed, he first needed to walk his talk as a scholar, and have faith in the earth himself, in his personal life. Nietzsche started to make long walks in nature to become as close to her as possible. Manschot followed Nietzsche's footsteps and went to the Swiss Alps and the Mediterranean Sea as well. He walked with Nietzsche and wrote a book on the meaning of Nietzsche's thought for climate change.[1]

Care for ecology begins with doing what we can in the microsphere of our lives. It also begins with accepting that we are entangled beings, entangled with our environment (Connolly, 2017, p. 10). We have less control than we have assumed. We need to rethink the relationships between the human-nature divide. On a global level, we need to acknowledge "capitalism as a geological force" (Connolly, 2017, p. 10). In the famous novel by Gabriel Garcia Marquez (1988), *Love in the Time of Cholera*, we find:

> Florentino Ariza waits patiently for decades to unite with Fermina Daza, and finally together, they essentially quarantine themselves aboard a steamboat forever sailing the waters of the Magdalena River. But in his zeal, Florentino, president of the River Company of the Caribbean, fails to see the warning signs of environmental degradation along the Magdalena. The "father of waters" is no longer the great river of Florentino's youth. It's been ravaged by 50 years of "uncontrolled deforestation," toppling ancient, colossal trees whose wood feeds the steamboats' boilers. Without these giants, the shrieking parrots and screaming monkeys have vanished, as have the manatees with their siren songs from the river's sandy banks.

## ACCULTURATION

Care is valued and expressed differently in different cultures. There is no universal perception of human worth, nor of poverty and pain. People die and people endure, and their communities follow tradition more than reason and reward. Economics, religion, and politics play a role. Even twins will not have the same eyes. Brinda Jegatheesan (2019) studied the perception of cows at her home in India, noting differences in religious and humanistic caring.

> Acculturation is a dynamic process by which an individual of a culture adopts/adapts to the traits of another culture. The extent of cultural and psychological changes depends upon the individual's conviction to his/ her native beliefs. Furthermore, changes within a family may increase conflict and stress among the members, making adaptations more difficult and complex (Berry, 2005).... I was conducting my research in the same town as my parent's plantation. Our family cow, named Sita, had recently given birth and was very ill. She was crying frequently and appeared to be comforted by her newborn calf. Dr. Peter (a U.S.-educated veterinarian, a native of India, and a practicing Christian), whose services my parents had utilized for a long time, visited the plantation every two days to treat Sita.
>
> Despite all medical treatments, Sita's condition worsened with time. Eventually, Dr. Peter informed my father that the cow was in pain and suffering and was convinced that she had at most two months to live. To relieve the cow of her pain and suffering, I suggested euthanasia to the shocking disbelief of the doctor. He told me that it was an "unthinkable act" and refused to do it. He repeatedly told me that it was a sin to euthanize a cow and that it would be bad *karma* for him. He also warned me of the *karmic* repercussions for me as a person of the Hindu faith. Even an offer to pay higher fees could not convince him. Unfortunately, all the other veterinarians in town also refused my request for euthanasia, and Sita eventually died 42 days later.

There are rules to live by, and rules so conflicted as to be unworkable. The answer is seldom to be found in the popularity or officiality of the rules but in the perceived hurt in following one and not the other. Or a mix or neither. The decision is an individual matter, hopefully taken as the different consequences can be imagined.

Rules to protect species and the environment are seen by many people as oppressive. The difference between the cost of giving up the old ways of living and improving the protection, in many instances, seems too large. The libertarians will remain opposed. *Compliance* can be a hard hitter. But others are changing and will change more. People and agencies can make the rules more tolerable by changing the orientation from *compliance* to *adherence*, sometimes arrived at through dialogue and negotiation. Adherence emphasizes shared benefit, lessening the feeling of submission and control.

> When Tomas sharpened the kitchen knives, which wasn't often, he wore a mask. He took care of his eyes. He was *compliant* with common sense and *adhered* to what his father taught him. Marie pointed out that the knives got sharp without Tomas feeling *submissive*, and that it's not what you call it but whether *taking care* feels more like "doing it right" or more like "being forced to do it."

The condors of California are not a pretty bird, scavengers, not seeming to do anyone any good. What loss is there if they are shot by hunters, and die out? Wildlife authorities were able to change some of the opposition by ranchers and hunters by free distribution of less-harmful ammunition. The care transition is shown in this report by ornithologist Mike Stake.

## Lethal Ingestion

Mike Stake, *Ventana Wildlife Society* (2019)

I pull up to a ranch gate, where three generations of hunters wait with their dogs around the family pickup. We have never met, and the condor decal stretched across the back window of my company truck will probably not win them over. But I brought something that will, and they give me a friendly welcome.

This is an ammunition delivery. Since 2012, Ventana Wildlife Society, a California nonprofit (not affiliated with The Wildlife Society), has been giving away free non-lead ammunition to hunters and ranchers to reduce the risk of exposing California condors (*Gymnogyps californianus*) and other scavengers to lead. With Pinnacles National Park, Ventana Wildlife Society co-manages the central California condor population, so it's familiar with the risk lead poses. While recognizing the conservation tradition of hunters, it has seen how condors may consume fragments of lead ammunition embedded in animal carcasses. Lead poisoning is still the greatest threat to the self-sustainability of the population. The hunters I am meeting today are among the 2,000-plus in the condor's range that have received free non-lead ammunition through this program (see Figure 9.1).

We sort through the ammunition I brought, and their questions turn to condors. The wild population has increased to more than 300 birds, I explain, with management playing a key role in that trend. The outlook wasn't always so rosy. Down to an all-time low of just 22 birds in 1982, and gone from the wild by 1987, condor populations have been restored thanks to a captive breeding program and releases by the U.S. Fish and Wildlife Service, Ventana Wildlife Society and the National Park Service in

**Figure 9.1**

*California Condors*

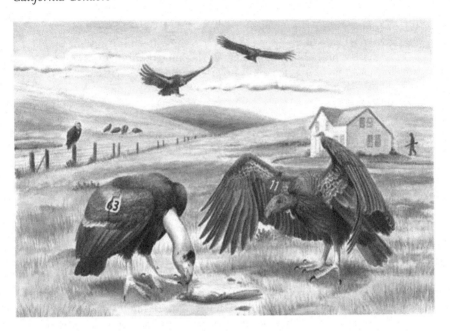

California; the Peregrine Fund in Arizona; and the Mexican Government and San Diego Zoo in Baja California.

The grandson stops me. "Are condors still dying from lead poisoning?" he asks. The words imply concern, but I detect a certain edge to his voice. We have observed fewer condor deaths from lead in the last few years here in central California, I reply. But, I am quick to add, lead poisoning still occurs and remains a threat to condor recovery.

This update doesn't settle well with many. It has been more than 10 years since the Ridley-Tree Condor Preservation Act required the use of non-lead ammunition for taking wildlife in the condor range in California. The requirement was extended statewide more recently, with full implementation on July 1. Some interpret the continued lead threat as an indication that hunters are not complying with regulations. Some hunters point to the persistence of a lead threat as reason to think there might be lead sources other than spent ammunition. These hunters have suggested lead paint or natural resources like soil, air and water as alternate sources of lead.

What is really happening here? With condor recovery at stake, it is important to understand why there is still a lead threat for condors even after the legislation mandated the use of non-lead ammunition.

**Small but Deadly.** The biggest reason might come from one of the smallest bullets. The .22 long rifle (LR) is a small round widely used by hunters and ranchers in the condor range to control ground squirrels and other small non-game animals. Because these carcasses are not typically collected by the shooter and are readily scavenged by condors, the switch to non-lead ammunition must include .22 LR to reduce lead exposure. This realization hit home for Ventana Wildlife Society several years after the ban in 2012, when its biologists found Condor #318 dying of lead poisoning. A post-mortem X-ray revealed an object in its stomach, which was extracted and identified as a lead .22 bullet. Ventana Wildlife Society does not discount the threat of larger-caliber hunting rounds, but there are reasons to be especially concerned with the continued persistence of lead .22 LR in the condor range.

It is not surprising that a condor might still find a lead .22 bullet when scavenging. I surveyed more than 200 local hunters and found that 83% regularly shoot .22 LR. But even though they are regularly shooting .22 LR, 74% of these hunters said that they "usually can't find" or "can never find" a non-lead version available for purchase. My hosts are glad to receive the 500-round brick of .22 LR that I hand them. They examine the box and pull out a few rounds, eager to try it out on the ground squirrels peppering the surrounding grassland hills. These ranchers have waited a long time for non-lead .22 LR, but others might be unwilling to wait if they have already invested in a supply of lead .22 LR. Rather than disposing of their lead stores at target ranges, where it is still permitted, some might be tempted to use it up on the ranch as they originally intended when the ammunition was purchased.

Local availability is particularly important after California passed the Safety for All Act in 2016, requiring face-to-face ammunition transfers. California residents accustomed to ordering ammunition online and receiving the shipments at home must now either shop at local stores or have their internet purchases picked up at a licensed vendor willing to complete the transaction. If most local hunters and ranchers regularly shoot .22 LR but are not consistently able to purchase non-lead versions, product availability might be having a substantial impact on ban compliance, and by extension, on condor exposure to lead.

**Adjusting to New Rules.** For hunters, the switch to non-lead ammunition has been an adjustment. The first adjustment for many has been the higher cost of non-lead ammunition. A few extra dollars per box might seem inconsequential to a deer hunter discharging just a couple of rounds per season. But, for a rancher dispatching several hundred rounds a month, the extra cost adds up. Initially, hunters might test multiple non-lead products to determine which is best for their firearm, and that trial process can be expensive.

Another adjustment for hunters has been gaining familiarity with the new regulations, not all of which have been clear. In the original text of the Ridley-Tree Condor Preservation Act, the use of lead for controlling small non-game mammals was not expressly forbidden, prompting many to wonder if their use of .22 LR for ground squirrel shooting was regulated. Some erroneously do not think of ground squirrels like the California ground squirrel (*Otospermophilus beecheyi*) as wildlife, and they don't think of controlling them as hunting for them. The California Fish and Game Commission later ruled that non-lead ammunition was required for shooting ground squirrels, but the decision was separate from the Ridley-Tree Condor Preservation Act.

Perhaps lacking clear guidance on the requirements, some were still using lead .22 LR long after they made the switch to non-lead for their big-game hunting rounds. The majority of my new contacts asking to receive free non-lead .22 LR ammunition in 2019 have indicated that they had not yet tried the Copper-22 brand—still the only non-lead .22 LR brand currently available. This slow transition to non-lead .22 LR is likely responsible for continued exposure of condors to lead poisoning.

Whatever legal uncertainty there has been, full implementation of the statewide ban in July 2019 brings more clarity by requiring non-lead ammunition for taking any wildlife— for any reason—with any firearm anywhere in California. As we meet with hunters and ranchers, we reinforce that ground squirrels are wildlife and are included in the non-lead regulations.

Even for hunters aware of the laws, it can be difficult to determine which ammunition products are lead-free. The Copper-22 behind the shelf at the local gun shop looks the same to me as the half-dozen lead .22 LR choices offered by CCI in their dark blue boxes. If shopping for the Hornady Superformance line of ammunition, in their attractive red boxes, a California hunter must be sure that it is loaded with the non-lead Gilding Metal Expanding bullet (or GMX for short) instead of the lead Super Shock Tip bullet (or SST). Both types are labeled as Superformance, and the boxes look the same. In this case, the key is distinguishing between two acronyms that say nothing about the lead content. Some manufacturers have begun adding a symbol on the box to more clearly identify California-certified non-lead ammunition, and this practice should help hunters make the distinction.

**The Key to Recovery.** Hunters and ranchers are the solution to condor recovery. Ranchers protect rural land, and these lands provide areas for condors and other wildlife to find food, water, and shelter. By switching to non-lead ammunition, hunters and ranchers are ensuring that scavengers, including bald (*Haliaeetus leucocephalus*) and golden eagles (*Aquila chrysaetos*), can benefit from healthy food resources.

But, solutions often take time. The higher cost of non-lead ammunition, the inconsistent availability of some non-lead ammunition, the uninformative labeling of non-lead products and the recent restrictions on ammunition shipping in California have all worked against hunters and ranchers making the switch.

With these hurdles, it is no small wonder that the lead threat still lingers following the non-lead regulations—at least for now. Hunters and ranchers are on the right path, though, and positive collaboration is becoming more frequent. The U.S. Fish and Wildlife Service, the National Park Service, the Institute for Wildlife Studies, The Peregrine Fund, the Oregon Zoo and the Yurok Tribe are just a few groups other than Ventana Wildlife Society that are devoting staff time toward non-lead ammunition outreach. This emphasis on non-lead outreach and collaboration promises to help condors inch closer toward full recovery.

After 20 minutes on the ranch, our conversation has ranged from condors, to a little good-natured ribbing, to some of their recent hunts. "My son here could sure tell you some stories," the grandfather tells me. I smile. "I'm sure you have a few of your own," I tell him.

They thank me for the ammunition and promise to tell their neighbors about our program. Perhaps their message will be that we really can work together for a solution, even if we do not always agree on everything. And while there is still work to do, teamwork on this issue is proof that we have come a long way.

## CARING FOR THE PLANET

Abraham Lincoln, in his brief Gettysburg words on the accomplishment of the Civil War, ended with "… that this nation, under God, shall have a new birth of freedom, and that government of the people, by the people, for the people, shall not perish from the earth." It rightly voiced Northern sacrifice in preservation of the nation. It could have voiced the nation's redefinition of care for slaves and women. Gradually we have come to feel differently about people.

And gradually we have come to feel differently about living things other than people. The social distance scales have meaning regarding animals and plants as well. Some of us are friends of chrysanthemums and enemies of crabgrass. Some of us are tree-lovers, especially the trees the power companies need not our permission to cut and those of the rainforest, and to most other trees as well. Our gardens and lawns and the plants in our windows should know the blessing of our care.

And even beyond the technically-living to those features of the earth which greatly support living. When asked about extending the priorities of care, Dannel McCollum, former mayor of Champaign, said, "Today, first of all, it has to be the planet." We need not decide what parts of the earth are alive. We can agree that the earth has received such neglect and abuse that it needs a better care paradigm. The well-being of people, animals, and vegetation, as well as oceans, skies, rivers, icecaps, and all of earth's stretches, need more of a care paradigm.

As book-writing winter ends, we join poet Ted Kooser (2000) in hoping his morning walk was keen and stretched enough.

## March 18: Gusty and Warm

by Ted Kooser

I saw the season's first bluebird
this morning, one month ahead
of its scheduled arrival. Lucky I am
to go to my cancer appointment
having been given a bluebird, and,
for a lifetime, having been given
this world.

Care can last a morning's walk. Care can drain a decade. The small and the large. The near and the far. The sweet and the bitter.

Many native Americans have had a deep respect for nature. Diamond Jenness (1930) was an anthropologist who, a hundred years ago, studied the indigenous cultures of Canada and Alaska. Musing about the Indians of Eastern Canada, he spoke of an Indian perspective of nature: "Not only men, but animals, trees, even rocks and water are tripartite, possessing bodies, souls and images. They all have a life like the life in human beings, even if they have all been gifted with different powers and attributes." Jenness felt that although man did not own nature, he had a responsibility to care for it.

## REFERENCES

Berry, J.W. (2005). Acculturation: Living successfully in two cultures. *International Journal of Intercultural Relations, 29*, 697–712.

Carson, R. (1962). *Silent Spring*. Houghton Mifflin.

Connolly, W. (2017). *Facing the planetary: Entangled humanism and the politics of swarming*. Duke University Press.

Denver, J. (2014). *Boy from the country* [Video]. YouTube. https://www.youtube.com/watch?v=MQoDs7EjiVU

Fineman, M. (2008). Vulnerability and Inevitable Inequality. *Oslo Law Review, 3*(4), 133–149.

Fitzgerald, M. (2019). Pluriversality and care: Rethinking global ethics. *Care Work Summit*, Draft Paper.

Hooser, T. (2000). *Winter morning walks: 100 postcards to Jim Harrison*. Carnegie Mellon University Press.

Jegatheesan, B. (2019). Influence of cultural and religious factors on attitudes toward animals. In A. H. Fine (Ed.), *Handbook on animal-assisted therapy*. Elsevier.

Jenness, D. (1930). *The Indian's interpretation of man.* Transactions of the Royal Society of Canada.

Kingsolver, B. (2002). *Prodigal summer.* HarperCollins.

Manschot, H. (2016). *Blijf de aarde trouw. Pleidooi voor een nietzscheaanse terrasofie.* Uitgeverij Van Tilt.

Marquez, G. (1988). *Love in the time of cholera.* Random House. https://www.sciencedirect.com/science/article/pii/B9780128012925000043?via%3Dihub

Obama, B. (2020). *We've seen all too terribly the consequences of those who denied warnings of a pandemic* [Tweet Post]. Twitter.com. https://twitter.com/barackobama/status/1245007713387544576

Rancière, J. (1999). *Dis-agreement: Politics and philosophy* (Julie Rose, Trans.). University of Minnesota Press.

Speech by Chief Joseph. (1879). In-mut-too-yah-lat-lat, Speech at Lincoln Hall in Washington D.C. *North American Review, 128*(269), 412–434. http://psi.mheducation.com/current/media/prints/pr_105.html

Stake, M. (2019, Nov./Dec.). Lethal ingestion. *The Wildlife Professional.*

## NOTE

1. Manschot's book will be translated to English soon.

# CHAPTER 10

---

# HUMANIZATION AND CARE

---

Nothing characterizes humanity better than care. Procreation, survival, greed, love, negotiation, and aggression compete for the focus of human nature, but care is always prominent. It includes self-care, care for others of the family, care for those of the tribe, care for animals and homes and gardens and properties. And the purse. It is often selfish care, but, overall, it will be care that requires endearment, nurturance, sacrifice, and respect.

Even without teaching, compensation, or legislation, care survives, but even with these helpings, it falls short of the need. Thinking of medical care and far beyond. There is no mechanism of church, state and conscience that delivers care to all the venues of need, and seldom in the amounts needed. The reservoirs of care are far from empty, but at a mark that needs topping up. There is need for care advocacy, a care ethic, to elevate the human mission. A care paradigm is needed to bring comfort and recovery more fully to the needy people and organic creations of the world.

## PERCEIVING CARE

Silence, please.
Please don't move.
We're going to listen to the silence in the cave,
and perhaps we can even hear our own heartbeats
Werner Herzog (2010)

---

What we are calling a care paradigm has long had attention by artists. In 2016, one of us visited Mullah's sculpture "Food for Thought" or "Al-Muallaqat," created by the Arabian artist Maha Mullah. It was exhibited at the Museum Voorlinden in The Netherlands (Figure 10.1). This work consists of Saudi Arabian long-blackened cooking pots that differ in size and that represent stories shared with each other, while cooking together. This lost heritage is a reference to the great muallaqat, or "Hanging Odes," canonical Arabic poems by great pre-Islamic or jahili poets from Arabia that once were hanging on the Ka'ba in Mecca (Malluh, 2015). These poems are about journeys of loss, remembrance and reflection, but also about "cultural understanding." To us, the collection of pots in this work, symbolizes the process of cooking as caring. Caring for food, for others, for community.

This wall is beautiful. Beauty matters to most of those of us who look in the mirror. It does, however, not have any formal position in our society. There is no such thing as a Department of Beauty (nor is there a Department of Care). But beauty matters to us deeply, personally, just like care.

**Figure 10.1**

*Cooking as Caring*

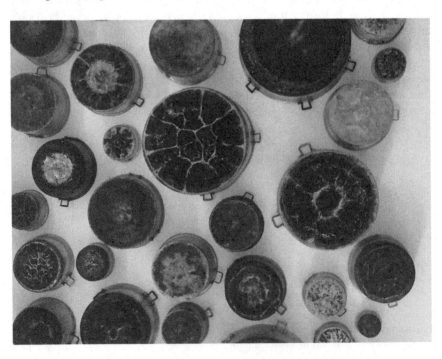

Sitting down, together with others, listening to a jazz improvisation or classical piece of music may lift us up, take us into another realm of existence that makes us aware of what it means to be human (Fernandez, 2020). The attentiveness, enjoyment and our senses bring us back to one of the most fundamental things in life: our body. The bodily sensorium, as some[1] would say, becomes alive when there is music around us that stirs us. When someone or something "moves" us in a sensory and emotional way. We hear, we feel, we see, we touch, we are touched, we may even connect to something spiritual, something that seems from a different realm than we can see with the eyes. In the 2010 film *Cave of Forgotten Dreams* (Herzog, 2010), three explorers went into the caves in the French Ardèche. Seeing the cave paintings had an intense impact on them. One of the archeologists describes:

> It was so powerful that every night I was dreaming of lions. Every day was the same shock for me. It was an emotional shock. I mean I am a scientist but a human too. And after five days I decided not to go back in the cave because I needed time just to relax and take time to absorb it.... I wasn't afraid—no, no, it was more a feeling of powerful things, and deep things, a way to understand things not in a direct *way.*

Care dissolves the boundaries between who we are, what we do, where we go. Care does not necessarily need to shock us like the archeologist in the cave experienced, but it can. It does not need to be powerful to our senses, but it may overwhelm us sometimes. In any case, *good* care opens, it lifts us up, no matter how much or how little. Living a care paradigm from an aesthetics view, is like being in a field that "holds" us like a nest, that leaves us free to reach out to others. Not out of obligation, but because we *feel* socially responsible for others. Understanding care may be an intellectual endeavor. It is also an understanding that is similar to the archeologists' insight: an indirect, sensory knowing. An unknowing, perhaps, of what we thought we would discover, being open to what is actually present. Here, and now, when we care or when others care for us.

Unknowing, indirect understanding, the sublime, and being silent are all values that do not match an economic or neoliberal view of society. People organize themselves around particular values: "You may share with your neighbor a love for orderly hedges but differ from his or her interest in literary prose. A good friend may like a painting you deem horrible (Pols, 2019). Aesthetic values connect people and disconnect them as well. Values run through classic sociological groups, such as castes, religions, nobilities. These values do not only concern how we look, or what we consider to be beautiful, true or good. Aesthetic values also distribute what we are able to perceive in the first place, *how* the sensible is distributed in our society. *If* we are able to perceive the entrance of the cave, its paintings in the first place..... Not how, but if. In the far past, it has been reported that no one was able to perceive the color blue until modern times (Loria, 2015). We could say that blue just did not exist, until some folks actually saw it. Blue just did not exist, until we knew. What does this mean for how we perceive care? Does it mean there will be new care in the future?

Perhaps we should mention ideology too, as it is closely related to what we are able to perceive in general. Usually, ideology is hidden, just as care can be hidden, but in a different way. The main character in the movie by John Carpenter *They Live* (1988) wears special sunglasses that unveil subliminal messages in mass media. In one of the scenes, while wearing his glasses, he walks in a busy street and looks up at a billboard. On the billboard, there is just one word: OBEY. He is confused: did the billboard change, suddenly? Then he takes off his glasses and sees a commercial for computers. A little more confused now, he turns toward another billboard, this time without glasses, and sees a beautiful white beach with a woman in a bikini. He puts on his glasses and the billboard changes to: "Marry and reproduce." Now, highly disturbed, we see him putting his glasses on and off and he cannott believe what is happening to him. We can almost hear him think: what is real, and what is unreal? He does not know how to respond to what is unveiled to him.

This broad view of aesthetics is no longer focused on art (although advertisements can be artistic). Instead, aesthetics becomes a form of politics that is susceptible to penetrate bodies, languages and institutions, operating through our everyday perceptions, experiences and events. The French philosopher Jacques Rançière (2004) wrote that aesthetics is not solely a matter of individual taste, choices or values, but also a matter of social and collective transformations that impact us every day. Going back to the care paradigm, we are surrounded by images, stories and other expressions that subtly influence our view of care. Some perceive care as soft, weak, and only for those who are a mother, or worse: who are vulnerable. Others perceive care as heroic, especially now in COVID-19 times, where care workers are visualized with astronaut-like outfits. Our visual culture of care can either promote or destroy a care paradigm, and everything in between.

## SOCIAL DISTANCE

How to respond to the need for care deserves one last attention. It is an art more than a science. We have been endowed with a gut, and its third virtue is that it helps us have a feeling for right choices. It is seldom all right or all wrong, but usually correctable. It is handicapped by having little idea of the total resources for caring. It surprises us that we can find another quotient of care. Sometimes Peter gives up what it takes to care for Paul, but we do what we can to spread it out. Or perhaps we seem stuck with what we do, and it is time to think more carefully about the spread. We will talk more about allocation of resources in the final chapter.

In Chapter 1, we mentioned the work of sociologist Emory Bogardus and his scaling of social distance (Bogardus, 1947). He moved to measure the general recognition that people were more supportive of others close by than others at further social distance, such as unknown people in other cultures. He used the following questions to provide a scale of separation. It was seen as an indication of the effort a person would make to give assistance and protection to others. The scale fits nicely into the notion that care will be distributed around the world less according to need but more according to affiliation. Pick any group, a nationality, a culture, a work group. When the yesses become noes, there is the boundary.

- Would you be willing to marry a member of this group?
- Would you be willing to have a member of this group as your close personal friend?
- Would you be willing to have a member of this group as your neighbor?
- Would you be willing to have a member of this group as your colleague at work?
- Would you be willing to have a member of this group as a citizen of your country?
- Would you be willing to have a member of this group visit your country as a noncitizen?
- Would you be willing to have a member of this group be excluded from associating with your country in any way?

Bogardus (1947) was criticized for too grand a generalization, but the fact is that we care more for family and close friends than for distant unknowns. His scaling is useful for us in thinking about whether our distribution of care is too open or too closed. The more open the embrace, the greater likelihood that dear ones will be neglected. The more closed the embrace, the greater likelihood of neglect of dependencies a little further out. In either failing someone dear may be hurt.

We cannot open our pantries equally to all people of the world. And we should not fail to share bread with those starving in the Sub-Sahara. We seek a resolution, even if it does little more than shade our at-times indifference. We are at the mercy of advertisements favoring one account over others. We try to follow churches and governments and philanthropies whom we trust and who seem free of corruption. We do little more than exercise our momentary sympathies. We should do more. And: we authors should have done more in this book. It is our aim to say let us increase the donations but more important, let us shorten many social distances. Let us increase each of our rosters of the care-worthy.

> Tomas and Marie had a difficult time relating *human care* to *climate change* and *animal care*. They didn't see it as having much to do with *social distancing*. They read some of this book and felt that the authors should have thought it through better.

## WHAT WORKS

Were there a perfect caring for any one person, it would not be the best for any second person. Just as no two persons are identical, their needs and openness to be cared for are defined by body and spiritual uniqueness and the uniqueness of each successive context in which they find themselves. Talking about both need and openness to care: It is not only shortfall in what the recipients themselves recognize as needed, nor shortfall in what the people around them say is needed, but shortfall in knowing *what works*. Any inventory defies a full listing, but each of the shortfalls and each of the hurts and each of the opportunities for being loved, each one stirs an awareness, and it is these stirrings, these feelings, that define the caring. Care Philosopher Nel Noddings (2010) put it this way:

> Care ethics recognizes the centrality of emotion or feeling in moral life. In this, we might trace our philosophical roots to David Hume and the moral philosophers who emphasized the role of feeling in moral motivation. Reason is required in analyzing situations and evaluating our resources, but we may achieve understanding and yet remain bystanders.

Hume (1751/1983) put it this way:

> What is honorable, what is fair, what is becoming, what is noble, what is generous, takes possession of the heart, and animates us to embrace and maintain it. What is intelligible, what is probable, what is true, procures only the cool assent of the understanding. (p. 15)

"What works" is a conundrum. What worked yesterday may not work today. What worked for five may not work for the sixth. For some, the side effects may outweigh the main effect. We have our theories and myths, and we should reward well those who study and respond to them, but it is a world of uncertainties. We cannot count on our experience or divinations to clarify the path. Still, we have no choice but to put art and science together, never excluding hunch and fear, to assemble a pattern of caring, for our loved ones and the world. Make no mistake, it is a subjective choice, but caring requires knowing something and doing something.

"What to know" is another conundrum (Hamington, 2018). We need to know the care needed at a time that no one else can give it, when the house is afire and we are alone. We need to know when the care already given is wrong. We need to know how to call 911 or a professional counselor. We need to get help, good help—knows best. Only a few of us know what works even some of the time. Most of us need practice in being dependent, not incompetent, but precisely how to mobilize a few who are competent. It is up to us to have a strong sense as to what could go wrong and where to find the competence.

"What to do" is another conundrum. In the immediate situation, one should be ready to do what the competent people tell us to do. From a Western movie came the quip: "Making ready: A glass on the table in case a bottle swims by." We need to make ready. They sometimes tell us to "Boil water." But that is still the water-breaking, he cannot get up, get-every-one-outside type of caregiving. Most of the doing relates to the long-term preparation for caregiving. Yes, still it's a matter of allying with the competent people, gathering date-valid supplies, and anticipating what could go wrong. These are not "do nothing," they are our first responses, the minimum level of caring.

They remind us of the poem by John Milton:

## When I Consider How My Light Is Spent (Sonnet 19 by John Milton, 1608–1674)

When I consider how my light is spent,
Ere half my days, in this dark world and wide,
And that one Talent which is death to hide
Lodged with me useless, though my Soul more bent
To serve therewith my Maker, and present
My true account, lest he returning chide;
"Doth God exact day-labour, light denied?"
I fondly ask. But patience, to prevent
That murmur, soon replies, "God doth not need
Either man's work or his own gifts; who best
Bear his mild yoke, they serve him best. His state
Is Kingly. Thousands at his bidding speed
And post o'er Land and Ocean without rest:
They also serve who only stand and wait.

Serving God and giving care are not the same. But the poem reminds us that we can be a part of the caregiving belief-system without being skilled in medicine or child rearing or any of the other technical services that people and other creatures need. They also serve who bring themselves and others to commitment to universal caring.

## DECENTERING AND CENTERING

The view of decentering is "bifocal" in the sense that good concentration on the task of caring is needed but also a peripheral view that draws upon restraints and opportunities. Microscopes can be invaluable, but kaleidoscopes have a role too. One should avoid being hell bent on care. The psychological term for avoiding fixation is decentering. By recognizing the centrality but not the complexity of our present perceptions and beliefs, we should see that it is possible to decenter them, and to be open to other arrangements. That is, we might have done better by being half hell bent on the care we are giving. The pace at which we have been going, may be over-stretching the family and other caregivers.

In philosophy, the word decentering is used more to mean bringing down, at least somewhat, the king, the human or the author or some other alpha, from high station. Thoughts about persons tend to dominate the interpretations of happenings; decentering opens attention to happenings that occur because of a culmination of events that we cannot control, or would not have predicted, because we do not understand their underlying connections. At the center, authors have dominated the meanings of words; in a decentered world social media might have more say. For example, the practices of "posting" and "liking" posts generate meanings unforeseen. In American politics, candidate personality has been dominant, in some more decentered countries, policy is the more prominent.

A society needs both people who do, and people who say. Saying and doing matter both. To not back up one's boastful talk with meaningful action, creates confusion. Luckily, there are many who walked their talk. Eloquently. We pause here a moment to think about who we would put in a Care Hall of Fame. Here is what we came up with:

## CARE HALL OF FAME (FIRST THOUGHTS)

| | | |
|---|---|---|
| Jane Addams | Martin Luther King | Eleanor Roosevelt |
| Jesus Christ | Bernard Kouchner | Theodore Roosevelt |
| Marie Curie | Cindy Levin | Ronald Ross |
| Harriet Patience Dame | Florence Nightingale | George Soros |
| Frederick Douglass | Sveinn Pálsson | Adlai Stephenson |

| | | |
|---|---|---|
| Francis of Assisi | Mary Ellen Patton | Mother Theresa |
| Mahatma Gandhi | Shimon Peres | Desmond Tutu |
| Maggie Jacobs | Ai-jen Poo | Oprah Winfrey |
| Chief Joseph | Mr. Rogers | Suzie Walking Bear Yellowtail |

But are we letting the media turn our heads to those who most visibly cared about care? We are omitting your grandparents, and the all-time human population of several billions, most of them spending large parts of their lives giving care. And how strange, almost at the closing of this book, to fixate on personal caring when we want to emphasize how care for nature and living spaces are just as important in a care paradigm. We need our heroes, our models, our greatnesses among men and women, but we also need to stretch our devotion to care beyond individuals to families and communities and cultures, and all the spaces and movements giving and needing nurture and protection.

Thinking again about the field of care ethics, what is rooted in persuasions, such as feminism, has loomed above the contractual duties of nurses and newsmen and women. Decentering could bring the several arenas more into common view.

With decentering, a care paradigm could mature into forces quite different from those at present. More habits, less rules. More impulses, less rationalizations? What seems unreasonable or unfair about the present distribution of care could be understood in a different light and changed. But it is unlikely to be changed through the old political, creedal ways. Different interventions will be required for care to be transformed. Ostensibly small alterations could lead to silent transformations (Julien, 2011). Care receivers could become more complicit in their service. It could happen because the political processes will be changing. It could happen when caregivers get more committed to a paradigm.

We have just spoken about decentering as a step toward allocations of care that would register in the minds of most of the people, raising expectations that there will be greater resources available for the weak, the dispirited, the harassed, and the suffering. And raising expectations also that all might live respected, in safety, with community, with fulfillment and joy. That, however-defined, may be part of the definition of the Good Life. Decentering the terrain of kindness might be one raising of the well-being across the cultures.

But we must also speak of *centering*, centering in a way common to the cultures we live in, particularly the culture of self-determination. Yes, of self-centering. We need to see a care paradigm as determined, as cultivated, as sculptured, by the choices that we make as individuals. It is folly to think that a new care paradigm could get voted in on the platform of a majority. Herd instinct is strong but is not enough to write the blueprint for care. It requires individuals.

Real benevolence is first the property of individuals, not churches, not charities, not governments. We have tried them around the world, and neither fear nor reward has done enough. There is little hope for education, formal teaching about care. The persuasion has to center on people seeing the need for caring further out, a little further, ultimately a lot further.

## REFERENCES

Bogardus, E. S. (1947). Measurement of personal-group relations. *Sociometry, 10*(4), 306–311. https://doi.org/10.2307/2785570

Fernandez, A. O. (2020). *La experiencia musical como mediación educative*. Octaedro.

Franco, L. (Producer), Carpenter, J. (Director). (1988). *They Live* [Motion Picture]. Larry Franco Productions

Hamington, M. (2018). Care, competency, and knowledge. Chapter 1 In: M. Visse & T. Abma (Eds.), *Evaluation for a caring society*. Information Age Publishers.

Herzog, W. (Director). (2010). *Cave of forgotten dreams* [Film]. IFC Films.

Hume, D. (1983). *An enquiry concerning the principles of morals*. Prometheus. (Original work published 1751)

Julien, F. (2011). *The silent transformations* [Les transformations silencieuses]. Seagull.

Loria, K. (2015). No one could see the color blue until modern times. *Business Insider Australia*. Businessinsider.com.au/what-is-blue-and-how-to-see-color-2015-2

Malluh, M. (2015). *Food for Thought Almuallaqat, 2014*. Art|Basel. https://www.artbasel.com/catalog/artwork/20610/Maha-Malluh-Food-for-Thought-Almuallaqat

Noddings, N. (2010). Moral education and caring. *Theory and Research in Education, 8*(2), 145–151.

Pols, J. (2019). Care, everyday life and aesthetic values. In J. Brouwer & S. Van Tuinen (Eds.), *To mind is to care* (pp. 42–61). V2_Lab for Unstable Media Productions.

Rançière, J. (2004). *The politics of aesthetics: The distribution of the sensible* (Translated with an Introduction by Gabriel Rockhill). Continuum International Publishing Group.

## NOTE

1. Such as Marcel Mauss at a lecture given at a meeting of the Société de Psychologie, May 7, 1934, or Maurice Merleau-Ponty 1945, Phénoménologie de la perception, Paris: Gallimard; *Phenomenology of Perception*, Donald Landes (trans.), London: Routledge, 2012.

# CHAPTER 11

---

# BANKRUPTCY[1]

---

It is probable that you recognize that you as an individual or your family are not distributing caregiving in the best possible way. It could be that you are overextended in some of your caregiving. It is possible also that you need some kind of bankruptcy procedure by which you could petition to reorganize your obligations, diminishing some of them, and get a new start on the help you give to those needing your care.

Bankruptcy would not be a good idea. The only person to receive your petition is you. And you would toss it out thinking that care cannot be commodified in the way property and debts are. Furthermore, bankruptcy is problematic everywhere, especially in matters of human relationship. Sorry to have brought it up. It was just too tempting as a chapter title.

## ALLOCATION OF CARE RESOURCES

But we still can talk about choosing what care to give. Earlier we expressed the hunch that baby care was favored over that for old folks, and that health took precedence over personal economics in Western society. Where are our data? We do not have any. It was just a hunch. It could be that the case-loads and the expenses for remedy are in a good balance across the spectrum. Our hunch says there's little balance and the imbalance is not a function of what people actually most care about.

---

*a Paradigm of Care*, pp. 133–142

The allocation of care resources is something we spend very little time thinking about. We do choose which charities to support and how much to read about the shortcomings of service providers. Usually we make our choices impulsively—distracted by the time it takes—rather than by deliberately laying out the choices. Not many of us seek out a *Consumers Report* or other sources to try to find out where the administrative costs are most reasonable. Impulse, asking the neighbor, is it for many of us. We are moved by portrayals of desolation, but those portrayals have little evidentiary quality. We cannot count on ACLU or UNESCO or Eagle Forum to point us to the truly most needy.

In this book we have said that energies for better care will probably have to come by getting more from the sources already giving. Along the way we add co-payers, more of them than we lose, but the participant numbers stay steady. Still, neither the old nor the new people can be expected to justify draining money from one cause to another. There is no triage, no justice system, that says some of our care for school safety should come from food safety. Such choosing should, of course, be left to the people.

But the people are impoverished for information. They know neither how safe are our schools nor our cheeses. Accreditations and use-dating are good to have, but the information falls short. And even less do the people know about likely results, the good that could be done if we supported Heifer International instead of Women's International League for Peace and Freedom, or vice versa. Data on all the care ventures would come at a high and controversial cost. So individuals and populations will remain information impoverished.

Still, it could be a useful few minutes to consider further the utility of that illusive information, were we to have it. Indeed, a little pondering might draw us toward furthering support for a paradigm. Rallies can be real. Recently we heard Alexa Babakhanian (2020) singing her composition, *Window on the World,* against a skyline background of Manhattan residents at their windows cheering on the army of unseen health-care workers.

Would that the streets of the world could be marched by kitten hats and face masks protesting the negligence of political leaders and vaccine makers and pharmacists who came into 2020 unprepared? It is a political matter. In the prior year, the Democratic candidates for the Presidency debated hours on hours without recognizing that the well-being of the nation rested on recognition that the World Health Organization and the U.S. Center for Disease Control needed White House respect. Joe Biden won the 2020 nomination not because he saw the need for appropriate response to disease but because he appeared most likely to defeat Donald Trump. Allocation of care resources is a political matter.

Our further hunch is that the existing care resources need substantial stocking, not just for health care but all care. And further still is our hunch that the leaders and legislatures and the mechanisms are not dividing care resources, including military and industrial bail-outs, in ways that closely fit the need and sensitivities of the people. The fact that they are elected has more to do with campaign contributions, cronyism, and lobbying than with their duty as representatives of the people.

In the experiential and material world we have seen three immense reservoirs of support. One, a reservoir of wealth, another a reservoir of human energy, and another of compassion. Yes, too simple, but bear with us. Three main reservoirs. We draw on these three reservoirs to keep the world's care flowing. The world's care-needs also can be oversimplified as three subsistences: health, property, and human relationships.

The oversimplification may drown us eventually but please hang in there a little longer.

The new question is: Is there, here and now, and will there be, several years from now, appropriate availability from each of the three reservoirs to properly support the three subsistences? If not, what will we do about it? Will everyone be housed? Will babies get more than their share and immigrants too little? Will protection of liberty get more of its share of spiritual care than protection from marauders? We cannot answer those questions. Try some easier ones.

Can we name three hugely underfunded subsistences? Can you name any funding that really ought not to ask for more help at this time? March of Dimes? NAACP? Heifer International? We cannot, with confidence, because we too do not have the information. Even the wealthiest, even the most blessed, even those run by the Mafia (are there any?[2]) may actually be doing the most good.

And where is the justice system that examines allocations, even by coarsest grain? The justice system is the public. Without better information, the people will make mistakes, but they should weigh in, with their support, with their impatience, with their intuition, as to how care should happen. How can we illustrate the imbalances so that they appeal to the thinking and responsibility of the people? How might we get people to the windows and the streets?

These are more than global questions, cosmic, universal, perhaps. We should not debate meta-philosophy while immediate care is needed just down the hall. Still, there is reason to think of whether the choices we are making among reservoirs and among subsistences need tweaking. People can do more than clap at the windows and march in the streets. They can speak out against the extravagances of pharmaceuticals and the sanctity of polar bears. They can speak more for care generally. A care paradigm touches close to home, and the palliatives need better recognition by each of us.

## PERSONAL ALLOCATIONS OF CARE

In the previous section we started to imagine how, across a care paradigm, the collective investments in care could be visualized and how we might better choose the most needy and justifiable recipients of care. And the only answer we came up with was: Let people decide in terms of their situations. Help them, but do not suppose there is or could be, an objective comparison of organized caregivers. Help them. Give them aggregated information on how total caregiving resources are currently distributed.

We may do no better with the question of, "How might individuals and families improve their 'annual giving?'" In a way, it is the same problem, closer to earth. They need to think about, talk about, what they already are doing, and not doing. "What did we spend last year and how much of our time did we donate? How could we be even better helpers next year?"

To speculate about personal allocation of annual care expenditures, we made estimates of what Tomas and Marie spent and worked at, to be helpers. We imagined a year when their two children had left home. We imagined one as married with an infant and the other in college. Both Tomas and Marie were working and their combined income was about $75,000. They owned their own home, mortgage free.

We treated purchases for new vehicles, clothing, appliances, and other property as not care expenses; however, repair on the house and depreciation were accepted as care expenses. Many outgoing donations were treated as care, even when the sums would be used for purchases that others would make of food, clothing, and household items. Taxes scheduled to be used for public education, infrastructure, and a small portion of military expenditures were also treated as care.

We classified the following main areas of care: self-care, health care, property care, charity, taxes, and education. We recognized that many provisions for care could be counted in more than one category; arbitrarily we placed them in one. The most difficult expenditure to classify was the expense for the daughter's college (amounting, if counted, to about half of the family's care expenses for that year). It would be a care for her future, but it is also a life expense. We decided to count it as the latter and not to include it within the care budget.

In this case for fictional Tomas and Marie, we estimated their monetary costs in thousands of dollars per year and labor costs in terms of hours per year. We treated their labor, their help giving, as a care donation at $20 per hour. (We followed the econometric principal of treating sheer guesses as thoughtful estimates.) Our estimates of annual cost for a broad definition of family care are shown here in Table 11.1. Some figures, such as health insurance and military, might be better thought of as availability of care —but still be treated it as provision of care. Taking care of their home and other property is care too. We pondered the finding that the expenses of care were taking almost half their income, $35.000 out of $75.000—even

**Table 11.1**

*Hypothetical Cost of Care for a Hypothetical Couple*

| CARE TYPE | Paid $/Year | Worked Hrs/Year | $@$20/hr | Total |
|---|---|---|---|---|
| _Self_/family care | $2,000 | 250 hrs | $5,000 | $7,000 |
| Helping close others | 100 | 50 | 1,000 | 1,100 |
| **Health care** | | | | |
| Medical | $3,000 | 0 | 0 | $3,000 |
| Insurance | 2,000 | 0 | 0 | 2,000 |
| Exercise | 500 | 100 | 2,000 | 2,500 |
| Mental health | 500 | 25 | 500 | 1,000 |
| **Property care** | | | | |
| Home, incl.depreciation | 13,000 | 30 | 6,000 | 19,000 |
| Equipment repair | 1,000 | 40 | 800 | 1,800 |
| Car service | 1,000 | 40 | 800 | 1,800 |
| Clothing repair | 100 | 0 | 0 | 100 |
| **Charity** | | | | |
| Church, incl. missions | 1,600 | 0 | 0 | 1,600 |
| Disaster donation | 700 | 10 | 200 | 900 |
| Poverty relief | 500 | 0 | 0 | 500 |
| Volunteer (soup kitchen) | 0 | 40 | 800 | 800 |
| Hospital donation | 200 | 0 | 0 | 200 |
| **Taxes** federal, state, local | | | | |
| Education | 3,000 | 0 | 0 | 3,000 |
| Roads, infrastructure | 1,000 | 0 | 0 | 1,000 |
| Military protection | 300 | 0 | 0 | 300 |
| Public lands, reserves | 300 | 0 | 0 | 300 |
| Mass transit | 300 | 0 | 0 | 300 |
| Subsidies, farm, etc. | 200 | 0 | 0 | 200 |
| Medicare, Medicade | 3,000 | 0 | 0 | 3,000 |
| Police, corrections | 1,000 | 0 | 0 | 1,000 |
| | $35,300 | 585 | $17,100 | $52,400 |

realizing that that half brought other benefits beside care. Few people probably would think they are paying so much for health, comfort and protection. So we should think more about it. We probably would think there might be better ways to achieve care from that investment. Care is not just providing comfort, it is sustaining life.

We then thought it might be easier to conceptualize if we represented the allocations spatially. We thought about a pie chart, then decided to work with a more flexible boundary. This made it easier to modify or add a category without affecting the rest. Here below we have spatial representation of the totals calculated above. If Grandma Marie began taking regular care of the baby, some space would change. And they and we face the question raised before, "Can and will we add to our care commitments without diminishing the care already being giving?" Surely some self-care would change, maybe the time spent exercising.

We have repeatedly emphasized the situationality of care. A budget for care is greatly susceptible to changing conditions. Or in different times and places. Were we to make estimates of care expenses in the Dutch life-scene it would appear quite different because of the social net for health and other human protections. And we would expect differences in Thailand. And between the mountains and the coasts there. And on this side of town and not on the other. Can we draw any conclusions? Perhaps not.

We found the distinction between life expenses and care quite difficult to make. Home costs are high here because Marie and Tomas cannot, by their own hands, maintain the vitality of their home. So they see it depreciating, and we have treated not taking care of it as a care. So, would rent be a care? And why aren't bread and water also a cost of self-care? We made arbitrary categories and realized how the picture varies with those choices. Still, we moved ahead, hoping to make something meaningful of the allocations. In Figure 11.2 care for the home is a prominent matter, deservedly so, given its guardianship over our lives. As the house or condo falls into disrepair, it adds to our need for personal care. The expense shown for helping others is embarrassingly small—then we realize that much of our tax payment goes to serve others as well as ourselves. And on we go.

These estimates surprised us. We already knew that county real estate taxes sometimes prioritize public education, a matter of care. And federal taxes go for the military, part of which we classified as a matter of protecting refugees. But everything military protects us—or does it? Public education is a care, but college education is a life expense—or is it? How we define care quickly changes the budget. The estimates are so arbitrary. The time Tomas volunteers at the soup kitchen could easily be counted as a contribution to his own mental health. So here again, as with the global allocations of the previous section, we are surprised to be reminded that many expenditures and labor can be treated as part of a care paradigm, self-care, and human protection.

All in all, what we see here reminds us that taxes, property care and health care are pretty much fixed. Keeping the house operative and making charitable contributions are the places where changes are available. But increasing the care budget is most available by cutting down on luxury items (not shown). Tough choices. How could Tomas and Marie be better caregivers next year? (Would you have been happier had we not ventured into metrics, hypothetical even? It seemed useful to us, but you know better.)

**Figure 11.2**

*Estimated Distribution of Care for a Family at Mid-Age*

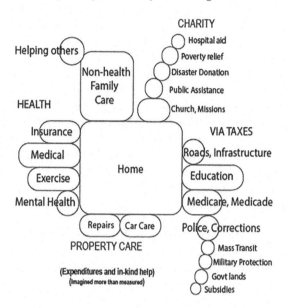

The urging of this book is to dig deeper into our own pockets and psyches, and to talk and behave in such a way that others are encouraged to do the same. We expect that almost all will think a greater care ethic is desirable. It is not always the case that paying Paul needs robbing Peter. Bankruptcy is not the answer. Nor rubrics to balance the care. The sensitivities are within us. When a baby comes, or a new tuition, or the next pandemic, many of us are able to shore up, to keep afloat, and to help a few of the many others who are sinking. The boundaries of care are elastic elastic and all too binding.

## COVERAGE OF THE PARADIGM

Let us make a last play with the concept of *paradigm*, not only as a grand idea or spirit, a disposition to give and receive care, but thinking of it as an earthly phenomenon such as an atmosphere or a cloud. Yes, it is also a cultural phenomenon, a sense of reality, a way of living, but we could imagine it to be a shelter or canopy. It is geographical in the sense that it extends over one to others, near and far. It is atmospheric in the sense that it has something of high and low pressure. The pressure is high where we care a lot, low where we care little. For each person this atmosphere has a different coverage, a situational coverage.

Society's grand paradigm is more or less the sum of personal paradigms. Each paradigm has a distance function; it extends nearby and farther out. It is changing, not as a cyclonic weather pattern, but as an evolution of attitude. For us in mid-America, we can think of it extending to Lebanon and India, where food and shelter and medicines are badly needed. We can think of the people of Puerto Rico, not getting the care extended to other people of the United States.

And we know a care paradigm extends beyond people to other living things and parts of our world. Beyond people. The cat, under foot, not getting kicked, is cared about. We have our pets and our chickens and our cattle, even when we breed them to be slaughtered, we care that they are fed and healthy and protected. Our care is not necessarily a matter of love and respect but extends to many varieties of getting others feeling better and avoiding distress. Did we whack the cat for knocking the lamp off the dresser?

But here we come to a particular social distance we have not talked about before. Clearly there are some creatures that at least some of us would rather see dead: rats, snakes, locusts, sharks. Not all of us are enthusiastic about keeping every species from extinction. Every leech? Every virus? There is transition across the map, often arbitrary, in flux, but a limit to the coverage. Thicker here than there. Here again the extent of the blanket of care is both a public and personal choice. It is not always easy to be more caring.

This book is not an advocacy of extension of care to all living creatures. The advocacy is to care for more than we do and to care better about those we care about. The boundaries remain personal choices.


## LOOKING BACK

Have we looked far enough ahead? Have we looked beyond the end of our noses? And back to recent and ancient views of care? This book's notion about a paradigm posed possibilities of including self-care, family care, care of those needing professional care, and care for the wide-world, all under the same cover.

We did not mean to make you think too much about this paradigm thing. It is the best concept we thought of for wanting to appeal afresh to your judgment of our commitment. Times past, we have been right in much of our caring, for our parents, sometimes for our siblings, for a few friends and the loves of our life. We have been too reluctant to forgive a few who have done us wrong, insufferable once in a while, tribal, too negligent in caring for the environment. And sometimes too reluctant to shed the shame for embarrassing ... who was it, you remember. Paradigm seemed a word as broad as ethic and belief, yet not mixing care with holiness and judgment. A paradigm of care, rest-of-the-life long, over-the-horizon spreading of care.

We have tried to make the point that care is partly defined by context. However enduring, the need for care is situational, a response suited to the moment, here in humor, there in tears. Who is watching, who is waiting? What just happened, what is next to happen? We are playwrights and composers, not in charge of the problem or the need, but tinkering with the response to the scene just ahead. That is the responsive thinking in caregiving. Here, in this book, we have wanted to concentrate on care believing, care anticipating, banking a firebox of care for times long coming.

For understanding a person, a congregation, a corporation, it should make sense to ask, "What is their care ethic?" For ourselves, "What is our paradigm?"

The easy part is helping get someone else, others, on station. We show the way, they come along, some stay. Stepping further is on the agenda. Mahatma Gandhi, the Indian spiritual leader, who perhaps had the greatest inclusion of paradigms, said this: "The best way to find yourself is to lose yourself in the service of others." Others waiting for the bathroom? Others newly unemployed? Others with homes in ashes?

We dare not ignore our own needs. The caregiver needs strength, tolerance, sensitivity, and humor. Happy relationships are built upon preservation of mind, body, and spirit. The nearest, then next, then further out perhaps than we ever thought before.

## CARE: A PRACTICE, A MOSAIC, A PARADIGM

In this book, our central idea about care has been this: Care exists amid standards, definitions, sacrifices, and emotions but should be known by personal feelings of what can be made better, particularly in immediate situations for unique individuals and societies.

There is no perfect care or pure care—it is situational. It is made up of disparate, sometimes inconsistent, acts, a mosaic of attentions, manifest in human strivings, responsive to the ongoing surround of people and happenings. Our stories from chapter to chapter have posted these views.

There is good care and bad care, certainly not indifferent to the wellness they accomplish, but essentially related to the practice of trying to make the immediate human condition better than it has been.

There is value in the views of disciplined and experienced specialists, but the views of all individuals are needed for the recognition of quality of care. What the cared-for person wants is seldom too difficult to discern.

And once again, a paradigm. A paradigm of care is the mind-set, the feeling, that care will be made available, with equity, to people and to living creatures and to the circumstances of their lives, as little based upon economic and cultural measurements as can be.

A paradigm of care is a resonance, a collective relationship of individuals with others and the world as a whole (Rosa, 2016), a harmony even among the atonalities of injury and suffering, predilections and custom, a widely-shared commitment to relief.

A paradigm of care exists among people with widely different experiences and values, even among those with contentious views of care practice and recovery but sharing the aspiration that the medium of caregiving be made better.

A paradigm of care is an expression of humanism, an increasing devotion to the sanctity of life nearby and afar, an investment in compassion, an attitude of benevolence.

All this, in appreciation, for what you do.

## REFERENCES

Babakhanian, A. (2020). *Window to the World Alexa Babakhanian.* https://www.drop-box.com/sh/z0csomkfbwvmbrf/AAC1_oqZMyVO4-einmUOy7Tba?dl=0

Rosa, H. (2016). *Resonanz: Eine Soziologie der Weltheziehung.* Suhrkamp.

## NOTES

1. If "Chapter 11, Bankruptcy" means nothing to you, our apologies. We are trying to be humorous. Skip ahead.
2. It is said some gang charities in Minneapolis feed children breakfast.

# ABOUT THE AUTHORS

**Robert Stake** retired as director of the Center for Instructional Research and Curriculum Evaluation at the University of Illinois. Since 1965, emphasizing qualitative research methods, particularly case study, he has been a specialist in the evaluation of educational programs. Among his topics have been: works in science and mathematics in elementary and secondary schools, Veterans Benefits Administration staff training, teacher education, arts education, development of teaching with gender equity; youth in transition from school to work, environmental education and special programs for gifted students, teaching in higher education, and the reform of urban education. Stake has authored *Quieting Reform*, a meta-evaluation of Charles Murray's evaluation of Cities-in-Schools; five books on research methods, *Standards-Based and Responsive Evaluation, Evaluating the Arts in Education, The Art of Case Study Research; Multiple Case Study Research;* and *Qualitative Research: Studying How Things Work*. In the 1990s he led a multiyear evaluation study of the Chicago Teachers Academy for Mathematics and Science. In 2003 he was mentor for case study research looking at the early childhood program of the International Step by Step Association in 29 countries. He received the Lazarsfeld Award from the American Evaluation Association and honorary doctorates from the University of Uppsala and the University of Valladolid. In 2007, from the American Educational Research Association, he received the President's Citation for work in evaluation, qualitative methods, and studies of arts education. In 2011 he was awarded the Career Research Award by the International Congress of Qualitative Inquiry. E-mail: stake@illinois.edu.

**Merel Visse** incorporates care studies with the arts and aesthetics. Her work results in conversations, papers, talks, experimentations, and collaborations that foster care. For the last 20 years, she came to understand about what is at the core of being human: care and creativity. She continues to ponder questions such as: How can care support us in living in a society with increasing demands on people and organizations? What is the importance of unknowing and mystery in the field of care, but also in the humanities, research and life itself? Creative artists are living those kinds of questions as leaning into the delicate and unsayable dimensions of our reality. Here, she works with philosophical traditions that explore an approach to the unsayable and incommensurable dimensions of life. Together with colleagues she develops a poetics of care research where phenomenality and life itself become the heart of the research. Currently, Merel serves as the Director of the Medical and Health Humanities at Drew University, Madison, New Jersey, where she was awarded the Meryll Skaggs Award for Excellence in Teaching. She is also an associate professor in Care Ethics at the Dutch university of Humanistic Studies where she coordinates the International Care Ethics Research Consortium. Merel authored a vast number of peer-reviewed journal publications. For details of her activities please visit www.merelvisse.com.